Veröffentlichungen aus der
Geomedizinischen Forschungsstelle
(Leiter: Professor Dr. med. Helmut J. Jusatz)
der Heidelberger Akademie der Wissenschaften

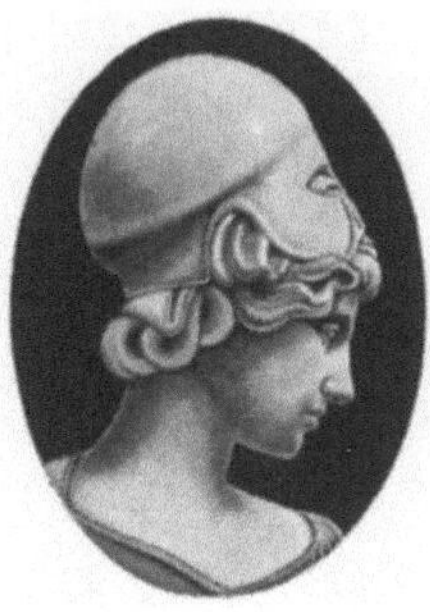

Supplement zu den Sitzungsberichten der
Mathematisch-naturwissenschaftlichen Klasse
Jahrgang 1983

Hella Wellmer

Dengue Haemorrhagic Fever in Thailand

Geomedical Observations on
Developments
Over the Period 1970–1979

Foreword by Helmut J. Jusatz

With 3 Coloured Map Plates, 1 Diagram Plate,
5 Text Maps and 12 Figures

*Submitted to the Meeting of 12 December, 1981
by Richard Haas*

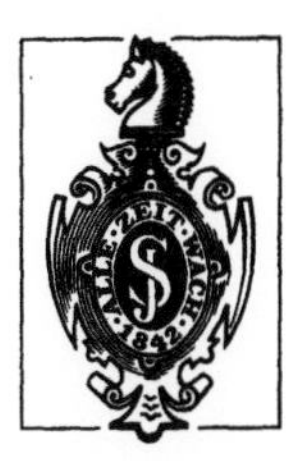

Springer-Verlag
Berlin Heidelberg New York Tokyo 1983

Dr. med. Hella Wellmer
Institut für Geographie
am Südasien-Institut
der Universität Heidelberg
Im Neuenheimer Feld 330
D-6900 Heidelberg 1

em. o. Professor Dr. med. Helmut J. Jusatz
Direktor i.R. des Instituts für Tropenhygiene
und öffentliches Gesundheitswesen am Südasien-Institut
der Universität Heidelberg
Leiter der Geomedizinischen Forschungsstelle der
Heidelberger Akademie der Wissenschaften
Karlstr. 4, Postfach 10 27 69
D-6900 Heidelberg 1

English Translation by
J. A. Hellen, M. A. (Oxon.), Dr. phil. (Bonn)
and Mrs. I. F. Hellen
Newcastle upon Tyne

ISBN-13: 978-3-642-69154-6 e-ISBN-13: 978-3-642-69152-2
DOI: 10.1007/978-3-642-69152-2

Printing and Bookbinding: Graphischer Betrieb Konrad Triltsch, Würzburg
Printing of Maps: Henning Wocke, Karlsruhe
2125/3140-543210

Foreword

On the occasion of a research visit to Thailand in my capacity as a member of the governing board of the South Asia Institute of the University of Heidelberg, I saw for the first time the severe clinical picture of dengue with haemorrhagic symptoms among Thai children. This visit had been made possible by Professor Dr. med. Dr. rer. nat. Ouay Ketusinh of Bangkok, to whom I wish to express my sincere thanks in this place. In 1972 the German medical literature – the periodical Medizinische Klinik, vol. 87, pp. 152–56, to be precise – had drawn attention to this new phenomenon in the disease panorama of South East Asia, indicating a change in dengue fever from being a relatively benign tropical disease to a form having serious clinical and epidemiological ramifications.

During the ten years following my first publication the new clinical picture, described as "dengue haemorrhagic fever", has become a standard component in the Thailand's system of notifiable diseases. So too, the World Health Organization publishes regular reports in its Weekly Records. On March 30/31, 1981, its Regional Office for South East Asia convened a special conference in New Delhi, thus emphasizing the significance of the diffusion of this new clinical picture in the states of South East Asia.

Hammon's discovery of the new serological sub-types 3 and 4 of the dengue virus during an epidemic in the Philippines in 1956 was followed by the spread of dengue haemorrhagic fever in Thailand from 1958 onwards. It has also been found in India, Indonesia, Sri Lanka and the south western Pacific. My original map, published in 1972, was carried forward by A. W. A. Brown up to 1975 and included in Melvyn Howe's *A World Geography of Diseases* (1977).

According to a new survey by A. W. A. Brown, dengue epidemics have continued to occur in the Caribbean since 1961. A high percentage of antibodies against type-2 have been found in the population. In 1981 type-4 was established for the first time in two American tourists who fell ill upon their return from the islands of St. Bartholomae and St. Martin in the Caribics. Dengue epidemics were observed on Guadeloupe in April, 1981, and on Dominica in May, 1981, caused apparently by type-4. In the same month Cuba experienced a serious epidemic caused by type-2: 340,000 cases of infection were reported, the peak being in the period July to September; it was also the first time that serious cases similar to the haemorrhagic fever type were observed. In January, 1982, a strain of dengue virus type-4 was isolated in a 32-year old man from Surinam who had never left his home in South America.

The extent of the world-wide occurrence of dengue haemorrhagic fever over the past twenty years has been estimated by Halstead to run to 600,000 hospital admissions and to 20,000 deaths. This author also recalled the existence of large

Aedes aegypti populations in the southern states of the U.S.A. − that is of the mosquito responsible for the transmission of the dengue virus. Downs has given an annotation in his Soper lecture delivered before the American Society of Tropical Medicine and Hygiene in Atlanta, 7 Nov 1980 that "our respected bellwether, dengue, has shaken the bell in Brownsville, Texas, in 1980".

To what extent the islands of the Caribbean and its coasts are at risk is evident from a world map of dengue occurrences up to 1957, published by E. Ulmann in Volume III of the *World Atlas of Epidemic Diseases* in 1961. This presentation, accompanied by climato-geographical data, has retained its value since it demonstrates the potential distribution of dengue.

The study presented in what follows does not seek to answer the question of whether the occurrence of haemorrhagic and shock syndrome linked with dengue constitutes a new disease, dengue haemorrhagic fever − the impressive phenomenon of which is, according to Halstead, thought to be based upon a particular constellation of dengue viruses of different types − or whether it is just an especially malignant form of dengue infection.

This publication is intended to draw attention to the new significance of dengue, which falls into the province of geomedical research and at the same time taking account of socio-economic and socio-cultural aspects as well. These analyses from a single country − Thailand − are not only intended as special research in the field for this country alone but, in the context of coming developments, deserve attention beyond that.

It is from this point of view that I wish to express my especial gratitude to the Ministry of Public Health in Bangkok which, by supplying most carefully compiled weekly statistical data, provided the basis for this analysis undertaken with the aid of the university computer in Heidelberg.

Heidelberg, March 1983   Helmut J. Jusatz

Contents

Foreword V

1   Introduction 1
1.1   The Virus 4
1.2   The Clinical Picture 5
1.3   Therapy and Prophylaxis 8

2   Thailand 9
2.1   Natural Regionalization 9
2.1.1 Central Plain 9
2.1.2 Western Highlands 9
2.1.3 Northern Mountain Ranges 9
2.1.4 Korat Plateau 9
2.1.5 South-Eastern Littoral 11
2.1.6 Southern Peninsula 11
2.2   The Climate 11
2.3   Vector Ecology and Human Settlement 13

3   The Dengue Haemorrhagic Fever Situation in Thailand until 1970 . 16

4   Study Findings 20
4.1   Material and Methods 20
4.2   The Incidence 22
4.3   The Endemic Area 23
4.4   Dengue Haemorrhagic Fever and the Main Transport Routes . . 26
4.5   Dengue Haemorrhagic Fever and the Urban Population 27
4.6   Density of Physicians and Incidence 30
4.7   Seasonality 30

5   Conclusions 32

Acknowledgement 35

References 36

Appendix: Morbidity Notification Card 38
          Notification Changing Card 39

Text Map 1. Dengue haemorrhagic fever, 1954–1981 2
Text Map 2. Thailand. Natural regions (According to Asanachinda, P.:
            Economic Geography of Thailand. Bangkok 1971 (in Thai)
            and other authors) 10
Text Map 3. Dengue haemorrhagic fever hospitalization 1962–1964 in
            9 health districts (According to Avril, 1972,
            cit. after Halstead, 1969) 17
Text Map 4. Railways and onset of epidemic spread of dengue
            haemorrhagic fever 28
Text Map 5. Urban population and dengue haemorrhagic fever
            (Population after Sternstein 1976) 29

Enclosures:
Map Plate 1: Dengue Haemorrhagic Fever in Thailand, 1970–1979. Total Number of Cases per 10,000 Inhabitants in 10 Years (based on Computer Mapping). – Dengue Hämorrhagisches Fieber in Thailand 1970–1979. Gesamtzahl der Fälle pro 10 000 Einwohner in 10 Jahren (auf der Grundlage von Computerkarten)

Map Plate 2: Dengue Haemorrhagic Fever in Thailand, 1970–1979. Climatic Regions and Endemic Area. – Dengue Hämorrhagisches Fieber in Thailand 1970–1979. Klimaregionen und Endemiegebiet

Map Plate 3: Dengue Haemorrhagic Fever and Medical Provision in Thailand (Based on Computer Mapping). – Dengue Hämorrhagisches Fieber und ärztliche Versorgung in Thailand (auf der Grundlage von Computerkarten)

Enclosure 4:
Diagram Plate: Seasonal Incidence of Dengue Haemorrhagic Fever in Thailand, 1970–1979. – Saisonales Verhalten von Dengue Hämorrhagischem Fieber in Thailand 1970–1979.
Below: Incidence of Dengue Haemorrhagic Fever and Precipitation in Bangkok, 1970–1979. – Vorkommen von Dengue Hämorrhagischem Fieber und Niederschlag in Bangkok 1970–1979

Back of Diagram Plate: Incidence of Dengue Haemorrhagic Fever and Precipitation in Four Provinces of Thailand, 1970–1979. – Vorkommen von Dengue Hämorrhagischem Fieber und Niederschlag in vier Provinzen von Thailand 1970–1979

1 Introduction

The viral disease known as dengue occurs throughout the tropics, especially in Asia, the Pacific region and the Caribbean. It is a general infection with relatively mild clinical symptoms, which is transmitted by certain species of mosquitoes. As a clinical phenomenon classical dengue fever is a highly febrile general sickness, persisting for 5 to 7 days and followed by a protracted period of convalescence. As a rule the course of the temperature curve is double-peaked. Pains in the joints and muscles, which gave the "dandified gait" that gives the disease its name, are typical. However, estimates based upon investigations into the antibodies indicate that the majority of dengue infections remain unapparent. This epidemiological peculiarity has been the reason that not as much attention has been devoted to infections involving dengue viruses as to those with yellow fever virus, although both of them are transmitted by the same species of mosquito, *Aedes aegypti.*

The early Fifties witnessed the sudden and alarming extension of a new clinical picture, which spread from the Philippines by way of Indonesia, Vietnam and Thailand to South East Asia and the islands of the south western Pacific, together with the occurrence of haemorrhagic symptoms differing from the process of an infection with the dengue virus which had been known hitherto. It was Hammon who, when adducing evidence of dengue viruses in the Philippines in 1956, established its connection with dengue. This was followed in 1958 by proof of the existence of the same type of dengue virus in cases of haemorrhagic fever in Bangkok. During the ensuing years dengue haemorrhagic fever (DHF) continued to spread (Text Map 1). In Thailand in particular it caused the greatest number of deaths amongst all the infectious diseases.

At an early stage a correlation between DHF and the occurrence of *Aedes (=A.) aegypti* was noted even if other species of Aedes were at the same time endemic in the area concerned. Only in 1903 had *A. aegypti* been recognized as the vector of dengue. This is in keeping with the altogether very late onset of work into the areas of mosquito distribution — indeed, this occurred only once their significance in the transmission of malaria had been recognized. It is for this reason that studies of the distribution of *A. aegypti* in Asia date only from this century. Nevertheless, all the authors who have concerned themselves with the ecology and distribution of *A. aegypti* assume on circumstantial evidence that this mosquito entered Asia only during the second half of the last century. Its arrival was immediately followed by serious epidemics since *A. aegypti* lives in the vicinity of man, prefers human blood when feeding, requires artificial water containers for breeding purposes, and avoids dense vegetation. The best environments offering these conditions are human settlements.

1
DENGUE HAEMORRHAGIC FEVER 1954-1981
AJMER 1969
KANPUR 1968
JABALPUR 1966
CALCUTTA 1963/64
VELLORE 1968
VISAKHAPATNAM 1964
MALDIVES 1980
MADRAS 1964
RANGOON 1970 1975 1977
LAOS 1962
HANOI 1958
N. VIETNAM 1958
THAILAND 1962-1981
BANGKOK 1958
S. VIETNAM 1961 1973 1977
MANILA 1978/79
PHILIPPINES 1954 1956 1966 1980
SRI LANKA 1966 1980/81
PENANG 1962
1977
KUALA 1973
MEDAN 1968/69
SINGAPORE 1960 1973 1978
SUMATRA
1978
CELEBES
NEW GUINEA 1981
MAKASSAR 1968/69
DJAKARTA
SURABAJA 1968 (1962) 1977/78
SEMARANG 1972/73
JAVA 1968/69 1973/74
BALI 1970
TAHITI 1972 1979
GFH

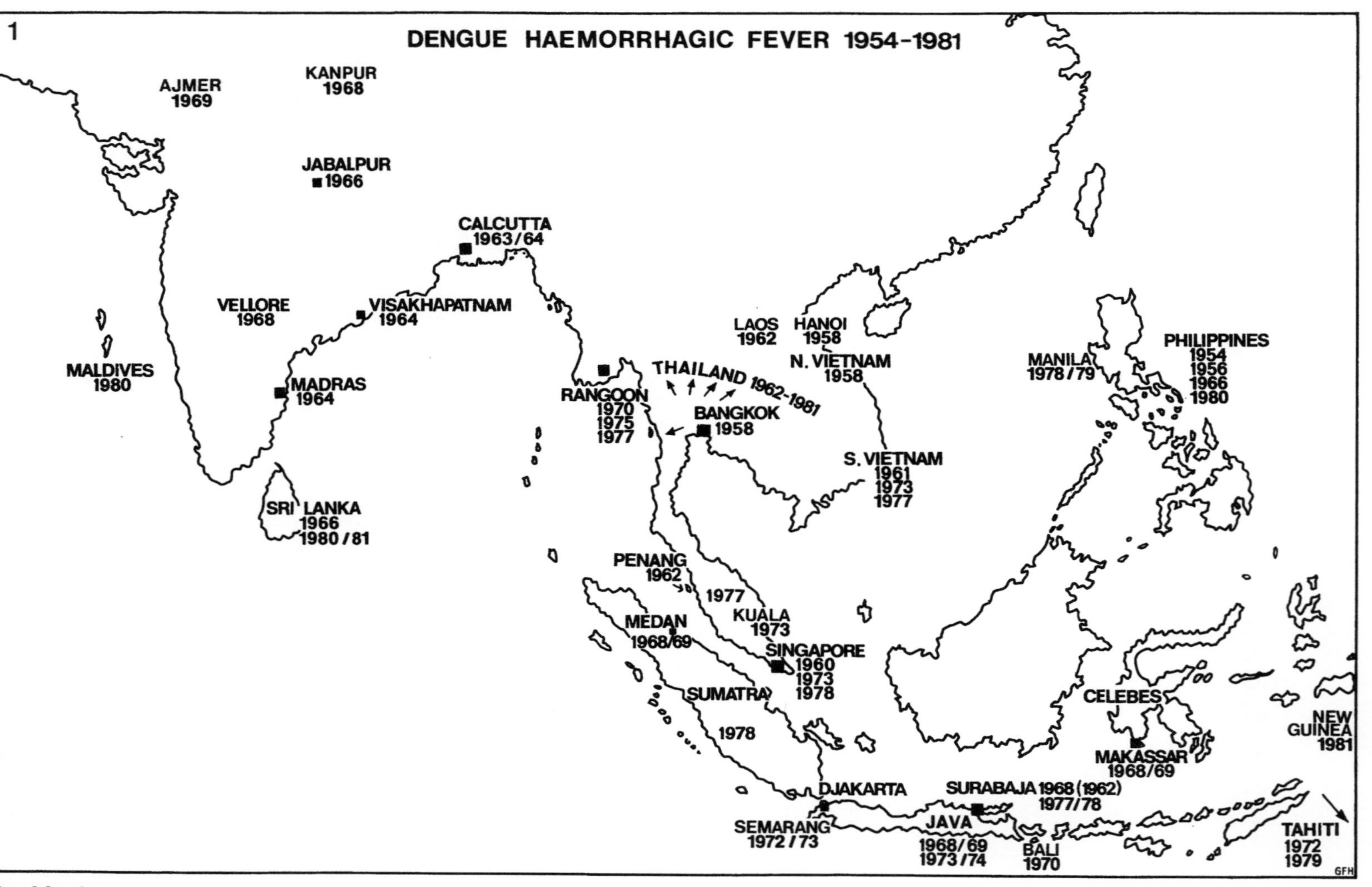

Text Map 1

It is significant that at the outset investigators were only able to detect the mosquito in the ports of Asia, the towns of the interior following later.

Gordon Smith (1956) developed a theory of the history of *A. aegypti's* distribution as well as of its penetration of the Asian sylvatic cycle, where the new vector caused a fundamental change. According to this theory the so-called classical dengue fever was originally a zoonosis of monkeys, transmitted by the mosquitoes of the bush. Wherever human settlements advanced into the forest so the *Aedes albopictus* mosquito became infected and in turn infected the people who had settled on the forest edge. In the course of time the high degree of infection allowed the relatively mild disease to develop into a paediatric complaint.

The development of large settlements, especially on the coasts, deprived *A. albopictus* of its breeding places in these habitats, since it prefers natural waters and bites only outside houses. The state of immunity in the urban population was therefore poor at the time that *A. aegypti* entered Asia at the end of the last century. As this mosquito is also an effective dengue vector, epidemics broke out in the ports. Such ports were the first to be affected because the eggs of *A. aegypti* are ideally transported by ships; they reached Hong Kong in 1902, Singapore in 1903 and Haiphong in 1915.

The urban population nonetheless gradually regained its immunity and after 1930 there were no further dengue epidemics. The disease reverted to being a disease of childhood. *A. aegypti* had firmly established itself.

During the 1950s a new clinical picture was observed in which the disease took a haemorrhagic course and ended fatally in about 10 per cent of all cases. In 1956 Hammon, working in the Philippines, recorded dengue viruses in these instances. As this, too, was a matter of dengue viruses transmitted by *A. aegypti,* the mechanism of this serious form was not at first understood. Even now there is by no means a general concensus of views on its explanation. Two main theories were advanced: the first was that of a mutation of the virus, the second that of a secondary infection by one of the four virus subtypes dengue 1−4 that are known to date. As most authors are now inclined towards the latter hypothesis, it will be briefly outlined here.

One epidemiological peculiarity had been noted at an early stage: only native people developed a haemorrhagic syndrome whereas foreigners who stayed a short time in the country developed classical dengue without haemorrhagic syndrome. Halstead (1980) reports only two cases of DHF in Non-Asians, both were children born in Asia. Halstead also describes how the graph of age distribution peaks twice (Fig. 1). The first of these peaks occurs during the first year of life, the second used to occur among 3-year old children in 1962, but has now (1978) shifted to those aged between 5 and 6 years. The shift of peaks towards a higher age is a well known phenomenon, which takes place when the rising immunity rate in a population is matched by a declining transmission rate. This fact can therefore also be taken as an indication of the disease indeed being a recent introduction. However, the peak among young babies remained the same, and it is obvious that a different causative mechanism is at work in this group. This was proved in the examination of antibodies, which revealed an immune response in most of the infants, as in a primary infection. In some babies and in older children the behaviour of antibodies corresponded with

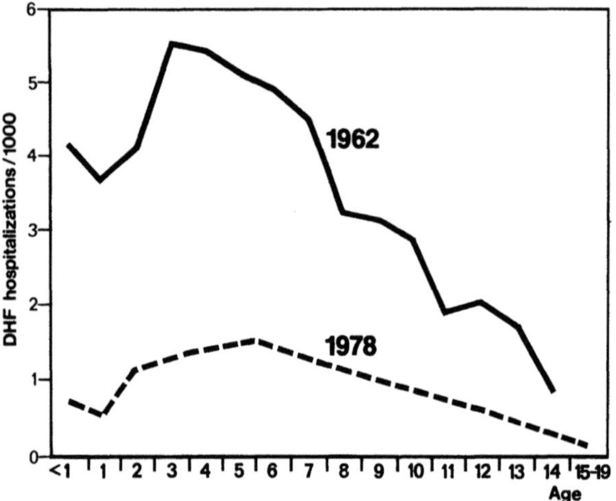

Fig. 1. Age-specific DHF/DSS hospitalization rates for metropolitan Bangkok in 1962 and 1978 (after Halstead, 1980); DSS=dengue-shock-syndrome

that which takes place in a secondary infection, however. Four sub-types of the dengue virus have so far been established; they are referred to as serotypes 1, 2, 3, and 4. All four have been recorded in Thailand. In this the body reacts to a secondary infection by another sub-type by developing the so-called DHF syndrome which, according to Halstead, is regarded as a particular form of immune response. Again, according to Halstead, in this connection it is irrelevant which of the known virus sub-types has caused the primary infection. The question of what percentage of secondary infections reacts with the haemorrhagic syndrome has so far gone unanswered. Mass surveys aimed at elucidating the question have so far remained unpublished.

According to Halstead there is an increase in the vascular permeability which consequently leads to bleeding and shock in the circulatory system. With almost every adult in cities like Bangkok having acquired dengue antibodies in the course of his or her life, it is probable that infants with DHF infection retain antibodies from their mothers.

Still it is impossible to predict the risk of DHF for the individual as well as for epidemics.

This study will not find the answer to this question either. But it may contribute to the understanding of large-scale ecological inter-relationships and thereby permit the prediction of DHF occurrence in an area known to have endemic dengue.

1.1 The Virus

The dengue virus belongs to the genus Flavivirus. Hitherto it had been regarded as an arbovirus (arthropod-borne virus), as this group includes those viruses which are transmitted by arthropods. In accordance with the new taxonomy of viruses now in force it bears the family name of *Togaviridae* and belongs to the genus Flavivirus. The dengue virus has, as already noted, four serotypes. Dengue viruses are capable of multiplying when in the tissue of their arthropode host. It is transmitted to the vertebrate being bitten during the act of biting and blood-sucking. The arthropod thus becomes a vector and transmitter of the dengue infection. The mosquito *A. aegypti* has been found to be a vector of both the virus of yellow fever and that of dengue fever.

The treatment of arboviruses as a whole from viewpoints which are more epidemiological appears to make sense in so far as they have also similar physical and chemical qualities. Nevertheless, a sub-division into different groups has been carried out. Together with yellow fever virus and the virus of spring-summer-meningo-encephalitis, the dengue fever virus belongs to a group which has classified as Group B. The epidemiology of arbovirus diseases varies greatly in accordance with the ecological requirements of its vectors, since a transmission from human to human is not possible. The distribution area of an arbovirus can therefore never excede the distribution area of its vector.

1.2 The Clinical Picture

Infection with haemorrhagic fever is a complaint of early childhood, infants and young children between 2—13 years, whereas classic dengue fever is a disease of older children and adults. For children of the age of 2—13 years there is an incubation period of 5—8 days after the infectious bite of an infected *A. aegypti* (Halstead, 1982).

In a typical case of moderately serious to serious DHF, illness sets in quickly with fever, stomach-ache and vomiting. This first phase lasts for about 2 to 3 days and does not have the appearance of serious disease. At this stage children are not taken to hospital. This is then followed abruptly by a toxic clinical pic-

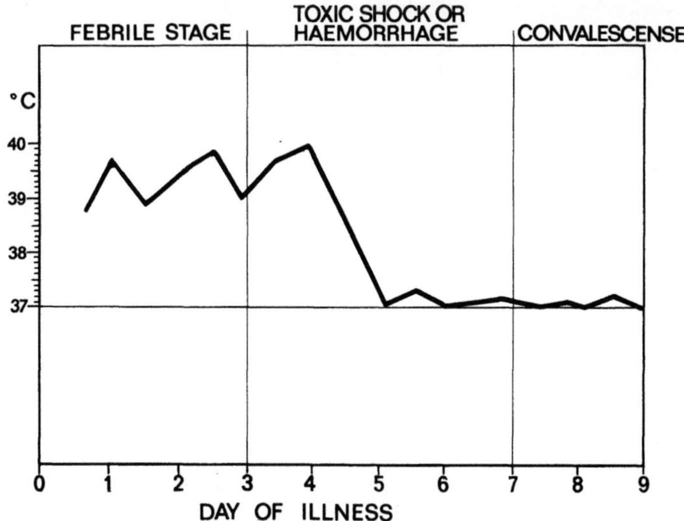

Fig. 2. Temperature-curve of a typical case of dengue-shock-syndrome (DSS)

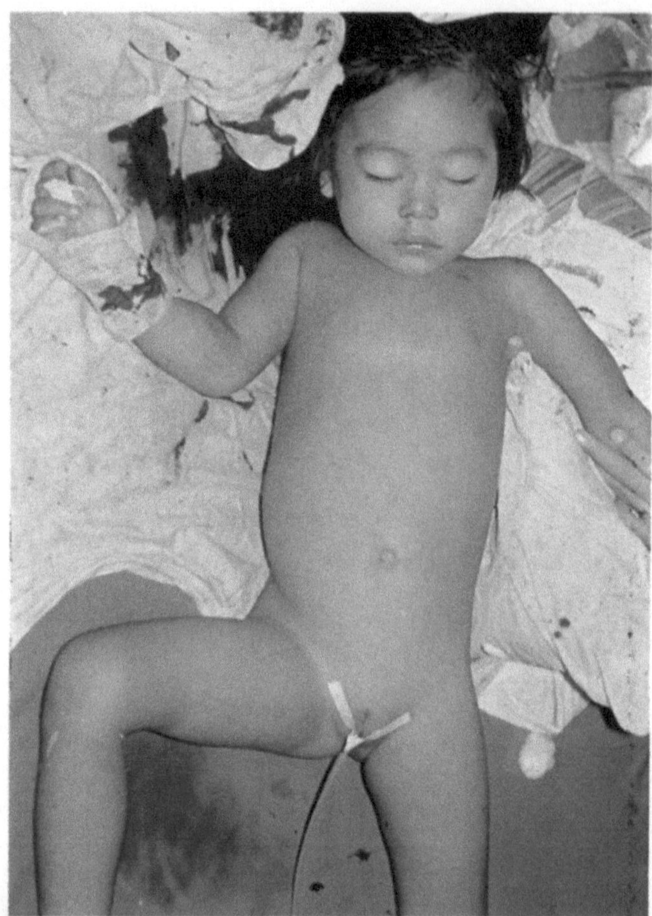

3

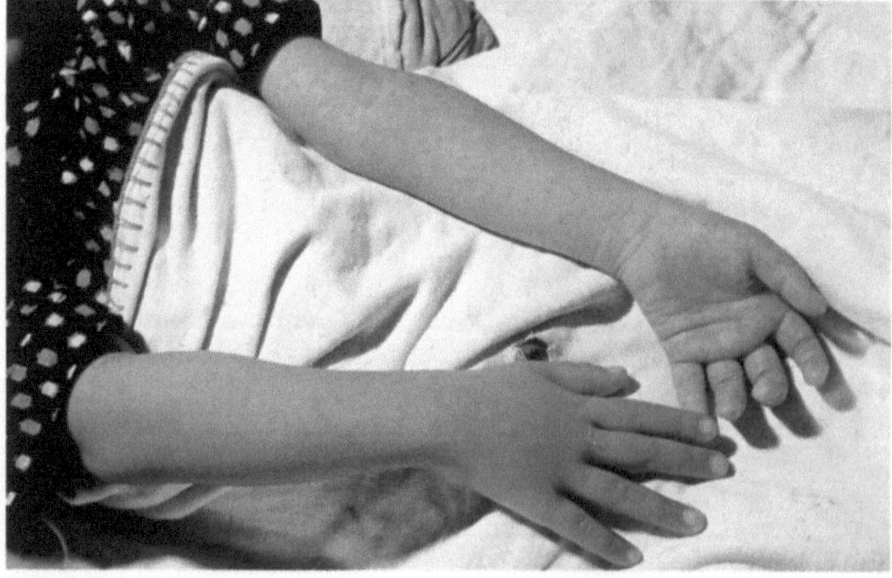

4

Table 1. Morbidity and serologically confirmed DHF in Thailand, 1978

Regions	No. of patients		% Confirmed	
	Reported (Morbidity rate) (per 100,000)	Examined[a] (% No. reported)	Dengue	Chikungunya
Central	4,278 (30.5)	1,066 (24.9)	63.9	1.8
Northern	1,644 (17.3)	591 (35.9)	43.8	1.5
North East	6,308 (39.7)	1,358 (21.5)	69.3	1.0
Southern	415 (7.5)	183 (44.0)	54.7	1.6
Total	12,645 (28.1)	3,198 (25.3)	61.2	1.4

Source: Dept. of Medical Sciences

[a] The serological confirmation of each separately reported clinical infection is carried out in accordance with standard practice in the virological laboratory of the Department of Medical Sciences in Bangkok with the CFR (Complement fixation reaction) and HAI (Haemagglutinin inhibition test). It is not clear from the collated data which method is applied in which case

ture on the second or third day (Fig. 2). The face becomes red and swollen, the extremities damp and cold while the fever persists. This tends to be the point at which admission to hospital takes place.

Shortly afterwards there appear haemorrhagic phenomena, such as haemorrhaging of the skin (Fig. 4) and mucous membranes, nose bleeds, or even vomiting of blood (Fig. 3) or passing blood in the stool. In serious cases a drop in temperature is accompanied by a shock to the circulatory system with the blood pressure falling below the point at which it cannot be measured. The shock is caused by damage to the capillary vessels, followed by a loss of protein and liquid from the bloodstream into the tissue. This stage constitutes a crisis point. If it is overcome recuperation is swift, occurring within two days.

Halstead was able to prove that a shock syndrome is more common in secondary infections than in primary infection (Fig. 5). But also in secondary infections only less than 50% of the patients developed a shock syndrom.

If there is no shock DHF cannot be distinguished clinically from chikungunya fever by differential diagnosis. Chikungunya is also an arbovirus infection with a course very similar to that of DHF. However, the climax of the illness already occurs during the first two days without ever incurring shock; fatalities are extremely rare. These constitute the reasons underlying the significance of the serological differential diagnosis for the prognosis. Among hospitalized cases the frequency amounts to about 1−2 per cent of the cases primarily regarded as DHF (Table 1).

Fig. 3. Child with shock-syndrome and haematemesis (photo: O. Ketusinh)

Fig. 4. Petechial bleedings in the forearms (photo: O. Ketusinh)

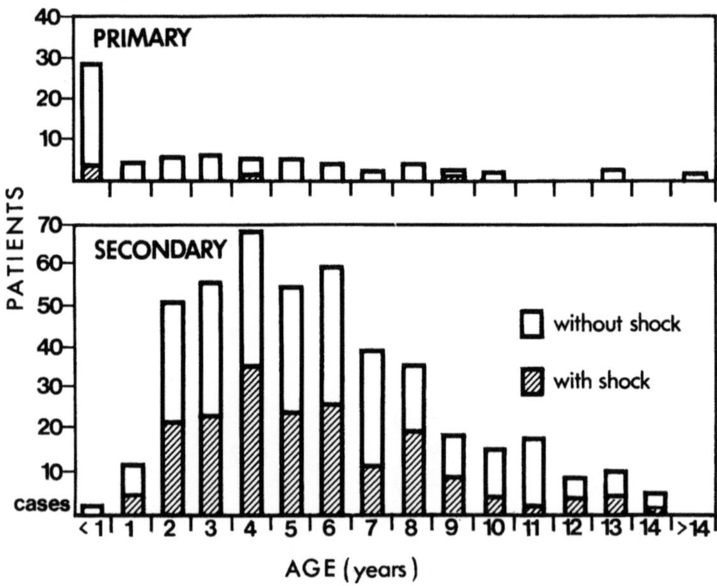

Fig. 5. Prevalence of the haemorrhagic syndrome with and without shock in primary infections and in re-infections by dengue virus, according to age (after Halstead, 1970)

1.3 Therapy and Prophylaxis

As in most virus diseases a specific therapy is not possible in the case of DHF either. Treatment is therefore directed towards the symptoms, with control of the circulation taking pride of place. Constant control of blood pressure and PCV (Pack cell volume = proportion of cellular components in the blood) must ensure the timely recognition of the impending shock and its prevention by infusion. The danger of over-infusion is particularly serious; in early times it frequently became the cause of complications. Restitution takes place relatively fast once the crisis has been overcome; the water which has entered the tissue during shock returns quickly to the bloodstream, thereby increasing the volume of blood to such an extent as to the danger to create a picture of over-infusion. If the problems of circulation can be overcome, further treatment presents no difficulties.

As is suggested by the case of other viral infections, a vaccine is being developed, though a marketable preparation is not yet available. The development of vaccine is under way at Ramathibodi Hospital, Bangkok, with the assistance of the Department of Tropical Medicine and Medical Microbiology, University of Hawaii.

At present, mosquito control must be considered the most important preventative measure.

2 Thailand

2.1 Natural Regionalization

The natural macro-regional units of the country permit the following division
to be made (Text Map 2).

2.1.1 The *central plain* extends about 500 km to the north from the coast of
Bangkok. It is a large alluvial plain rising only a few metres above sea-level and
subject to annual flooding. It is dissected by innumerable canals and rivers, the
largest of which is the Chaophaya Menam. It is a densely settled and agricul-
turally intensively utilized region. By far the greatest part of the central plain is
situated in Thailand's arid climatic region.

2.1.2 In the west the central plain is bounded by the *western highlands* forming
the border with Burma.

2.1.3 The *northern mountain ranges* are the part of the country to the north of
the central plain. Running from north to south, the densely forested mountain
ranges include numerous valleys, the broader ones of which are used agricultur-
ally. The hill tribes are shifting cultivators who clear plots by burning. They
have only limited contact with the Thai population.

Further south the rivers of the valleys join the spring waters of the Chaophaya Menam, apart from the most distant north west, which drains to the
Salween, and the furthest north, which drains towards the Mekong. The mountains of northern Thailand reach maximum altitudes of 2,595 m above sea-
level. The climate is a humid one, totalling 6.5 to 8 humid months a year, with
valleys remaining somewhat drier. During the winter months the mean monthly
temperature falls below 22 °C for about 1 to 3 months a year, a fact not without
significance for the development cycle of *A. aegypti.*

2.1.4 The *Korat Plateau* in eastern Thailand is a shallow basin situated at an
altitude of 130−170 m above sea-level occupying a distinctly higher level than
the central plain; in the west and south it is surrounded by a rim of hills reaching heights from several hundred to 1,700 metres. In the east the Korat Plateau
is bounded by the Mekong, which forms the political border with Laos at the
same time.

With a mere 4.5 to 5.5 humid months a year, the climate in the centre of the
Korat Plateau is very dry, although large tracts of land are flooded during the
rainy season, or turn into swamp. Considering the year as a whole, the eastern

2
THAILAND
NATURAL REGIONS
I
NORTHERN MOUNTAIN RANGES
II
WESTERN HIGHLANDS
III
CENTRAL PLAIN
IV
KORAT PLATEAU
(= EASTERN PLAINS AND MOUNTAINS)
V
SOUTHEASTERN LITTORAL
VI
SOUTHERN PENINSULA
GFH.
20°
18°
16°
14°
12°
10°
8°
98°
100°
102°
104°

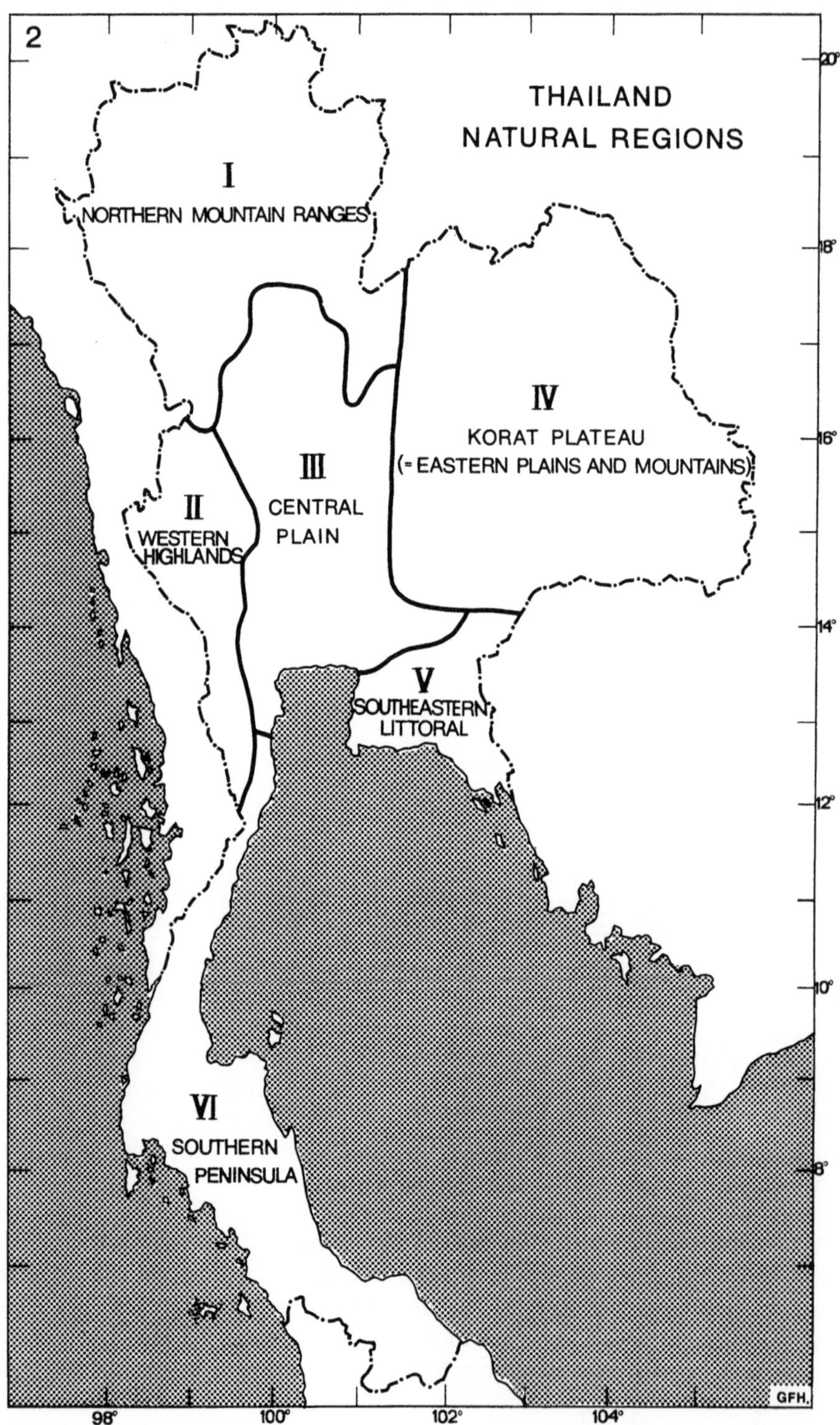

Text Map 2

areas of Korat Plateau regions are wetter than the western parts, though they receive their precipitation exclusively during the summer monsoon.

Apart from the population concentrations in the cities, the Korat Plateau is sparsely settled.

2.1.5 South-eastern littoral follows directly upon the population centres of the central plain and even ten years ago it had a relatively high proportion of urban population which made up ten per cent of the total.

With the outliers of the Cardamom Mountains the most south-easterly part is situated in the realm of the permanently humid tropics.

2.1.6 The *southern peninsula* occupies part of the Malayan peninsula. In places where this strip borders on Burma, it is locally only 20 km wide. Running in a north to south direction, the central mountains divide Southern Thailand into an eastern section, facing the Gulf of Siam and thus the north east monsoon, and a western part receiving the south west monsoon. But in spite of the monsoonal differences in precipitation, atmospheric humidity remains high throughout the year since southern Thailand is situated in the permanently humid tropical realm.

2.2 The Climate

Thailand lies in the zone of influence of the monsoons which determine the amount and the distribution of precipitation all over the country. Apart from

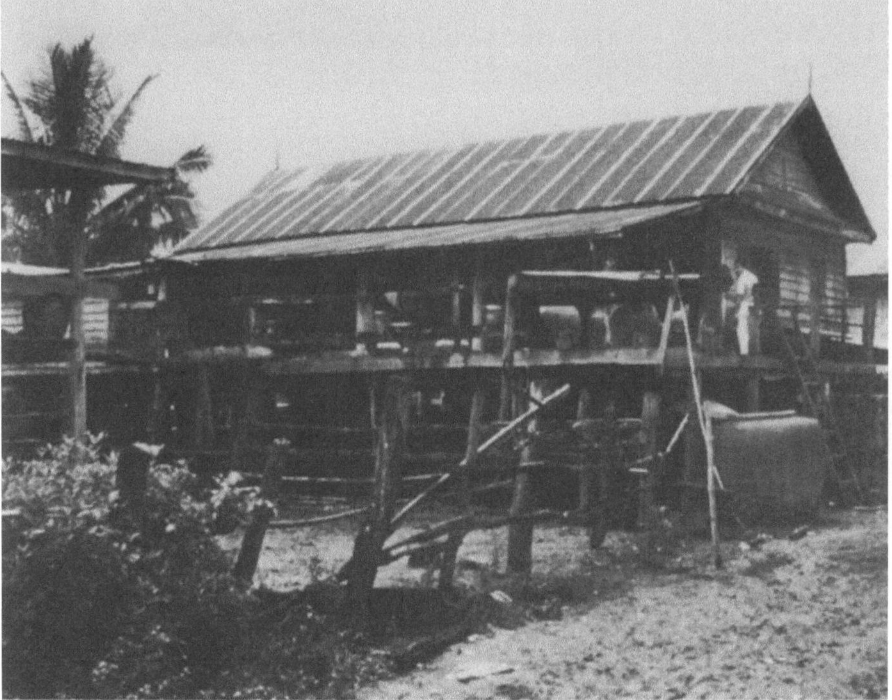

Fig. 6. Village house in Nong Waeng, Province of Khon Kaen (photo: H. Wellmer)

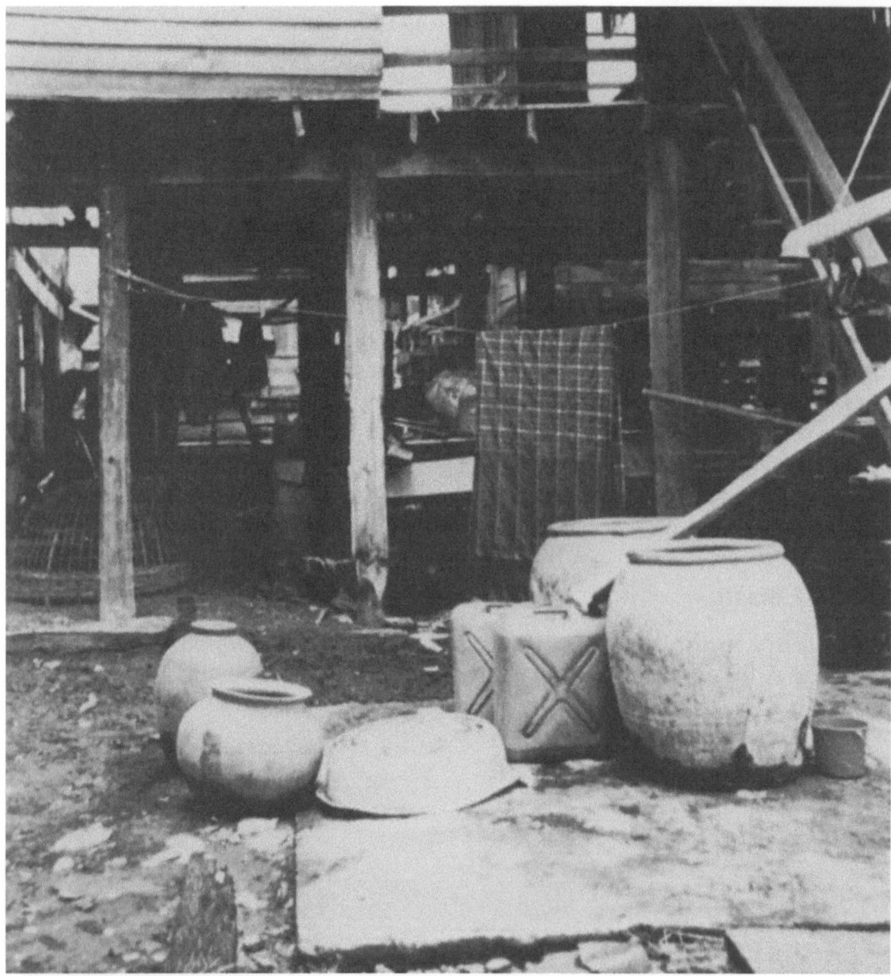

Fig. 7. Water containers collecting rain water from the roof (photo: H. Wellmer)

the east coast of the southern peninsula, the south west monsoon is the chief bringer of rain (May—Sept.). Above all it carries rain to those parts of the country which are near the mountains, whereas in the centre of the country evaporation exceeds precipitation during most months of the year (Map Plate 2).

Temperatures are high throughout the year, with monthly averages ranging between 22 °C and 30 °C except in northern Thailand, where the temperature may fall below 22 °C and even to 16 °C (Chiang Rai) during the period November to January, the winter months. These low temperatures are the condition of the northern limit of *A. aegypti*. This mosquito will stop its development cycle when temperatures drop below 20 °C (Aiken, 1977). Under the conditions of only 1—3 months with low temperatures, *A. aegypti* will survive but its population number will be kept low. Occasionally monthly averages of less than 22 °C are also recorded in the north of the Korat Plateau to the north of the 16th parallel during December and January.

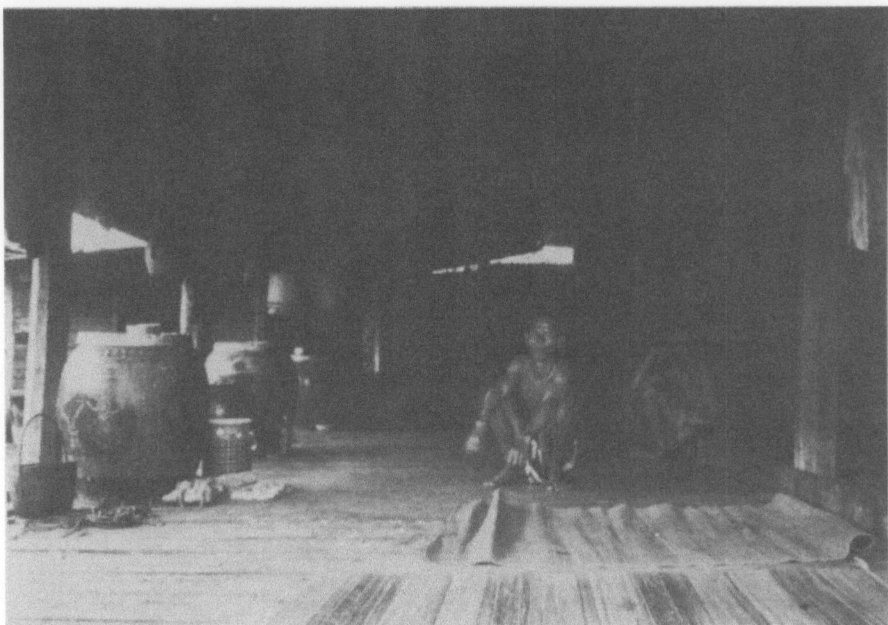

Fig. 8. Open verandah and water containers (photo: H. Wellmer)

2.3 Vector Ecology and Human Settlement

Wherever man has altered the environment he has done so in favour of
A. aegypti, the vector of dengue. It is therefore not surprising that it occurs in
particularly large numbers in the vicinity of human settlements.

In South East Asia, and thus in Thailand too, a population explosion and
rapid growth of cities led to a deterioration in sanitary conditions. The re-
duction of vegetation and shade outside houses, together with an increase in
man-made containers for drinking water enhanced the breeding possibilities for
A. aegypti whilst, at the same time, changing them for the worse for *A. albopictus*, the autochtonous vector, which has almost disappeared from Bangkok.

Pant (1973) was able to establish that in a Breteau index[1] below 20 very few
cases of DHF were found, whereas many more occurred in a Breteau index of
more than 50, and 69–153 were counted in epidemic areas at the time of the
1971 epidemic. The vessels listed by him included large and small containers
that happened to be filled with water, as well as traditional earthenware storage
jars with capacities of up to 200 litres.

At Saraburi, for example, a provincial capital about 100 km from Bangkok,
the average quantity of water stored per house amounted to 180–200 litres
(WHO Weekly, 1971). The reason for this was said to be the particularly poor
urban water supply there, which makes the tradition a necessity. Rainwater collected on roofs and led into giant containers by way of a system of gutters, is
generally preferred as drinking water (Figs. 6 and 7). Their size prevents these

---

[1] Number of positive containers per 100 houses

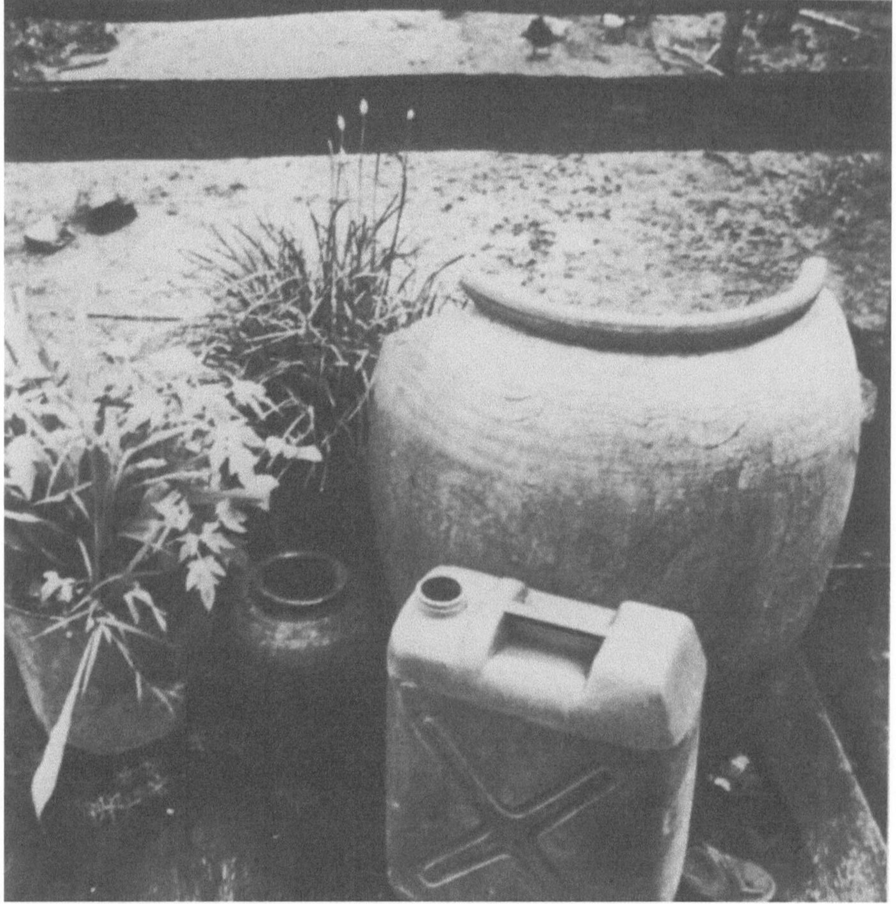

Fig. 9. Not used tins and pots in a garden (photo: H. Wellmer)

containers from being moved and they remain as near as possible to the house (Fig. 8). Water for general use is taken from the river or other waters. Containers used for this are emptied much more regularly, a fact which makes them less likely breeding places for mosquitoes.

The average number of possible breeding places per house at Saraburi was 9.3, but not all the containers proved to be positive: the container index[2] amounted to 52.7 – a still high enough figure, of course.

The female of *A. aegypti* deposits her eggs on a container wall a little above the surface of the water – i.e. to start with a container with a wall above a water surface is all that is required. When the water level rises as a result of rain, for example, the eggs are wetted. Within a few hours the larvae hatch and become fully adult within a matter of a few days.

---

[2] Number of larvae-positive water holding containers per 100 containers

In this way not only do water containers offer ideal developmental conditions to the dengue vectors, they furnish food supplies in the immediate vicinity as well, that is man himself, the blood of whom *A. aegypti* prefers to that of all other vertebrates. The density of infestation is indicated by the house index, i.e. the percentage of positively affected houses for *A. aegypti*. Earthenware jars are not the only ones to be used as breeding places. To these must also be added especially the water containers placed at the foot of furniture so as to trap ants and never emptied, and of course every can that has been thrown aside, every old car tyre and all other refuse capable of filling with water when it rains (Fig. 9). All the breeding places have one thing in common: they occur as a result of, and in the vicinity of, human settlements.

In the ten year period from 1960 to 1970 Bangkok had grown from a population of 2.1 million to one of 3.5 million; one third of its 1970 extent of 285 km² was covered by slums (Donner, 1972). Since then the residential population has experienced an annual increase of 7 per cent. At the same time other urban centres elsewhere in the country also underwent an accelerated development, including intensified contruction of transport routes.

3 The Dengue Haemorrhagic Fever Situation in Thailand Until 1970

In 1958 when − on the occasion of the first epidemic with more than 2,000 cases in Bangkok − the serological and virological proof was obtained which established that dengue viruses were involved, a haemorrhagic fever syndrome had not been entirely unknown in Bangkok (personal cummunication from Prof. Direk Pongpipat, Siriraj Hospital, Bangkok).

Until 1960 DHF was practically limited to the urban area proper, spreading to the outer districts and adjoining provinces during the ensuing two years, and being reported from all the larger centres of population of the country by 1962. At that time registration took place within the context of the nine health regions. However, the extent of their involvement varied greatly (Table 2 and Text Map 3).

The provincial capitals, which were the first to be affected, are located along the major railway lines (see Text Map 4). This fact is in accordance with McDonald's statement in terms of which railways make an ideal transport mode for the eggs of *A. aegypti*.

In 1968 Mae Hong Son, Krabi, Satun and Trang were the only four provinces not to have reported a single case of DHF. Even now these provinces continue to report a very small number of cases.

Until 1968 it looked as if DHF was set to increase and decrease in a two-year rhythm, but the then highest number of 6,032 reported cases was followed by a previously unmatched epidemic extent in 1969 involving 8,613 recorded infections (see Table 3). Since then the two-year rhythm has become blurred (Fig. 10).

Table 2. Dengue haemorrhagic fever hospitalization in the 9 health districts of Thailand during the period 1962−1964 (from Avril, 1972, quoted by Halstead, 1969)

	1962	1963	1964	total
I	327	200	939	1,466
II	588	468	720	1,776
III	22	23	1,018	1,063
IV	8	2	188	198
V	3	15	276	294
VI	656	430	233	1,319
VII	646	592	579	1,817
VIII	66	26	82	174
IX	2	11	4	17

3
Dengue haemorrhagic fever
hospitalization 1962-1964
in 9 health districts
cases:
0 - 101
101 - 1000
1001 - 1400
1401 - 1900
0   50   100
Km
GFH

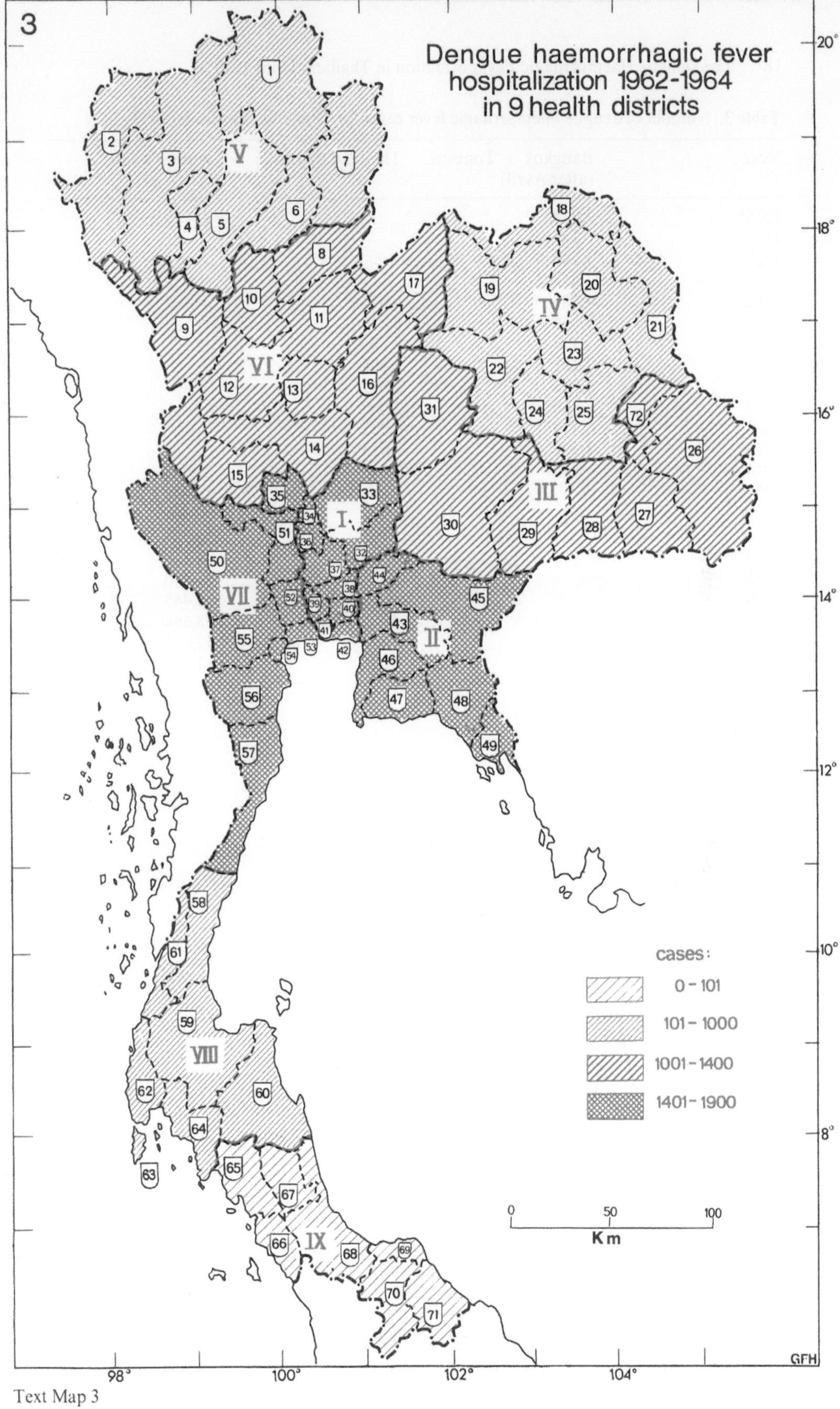

Text Map 3

Table 3. Number of dengue haemorrhagic fever cases for Thailand as a whole, 1958–1979

Year	Bangkok + Tonburi (after Avril)	Thailand in toto	Author's data
1958	2,418		
1959	127		
1960	1,742		
1961	418		
1962	4,187	6,078	
1963	1,644	3,070	
1964	5,358	9,020	
1965	1,253	3,466	
1966	1,986	5,845	
1967	358	2,060	
1968	779	6,032	
1969	1,385	8,613	
1970	574	2,840	2,743
1971			11,296
1972			23,560
1973			8,283
1974			8,112
1975			17,440
1976			9,445
1977			38,664
1978			12,042
1979			11,412

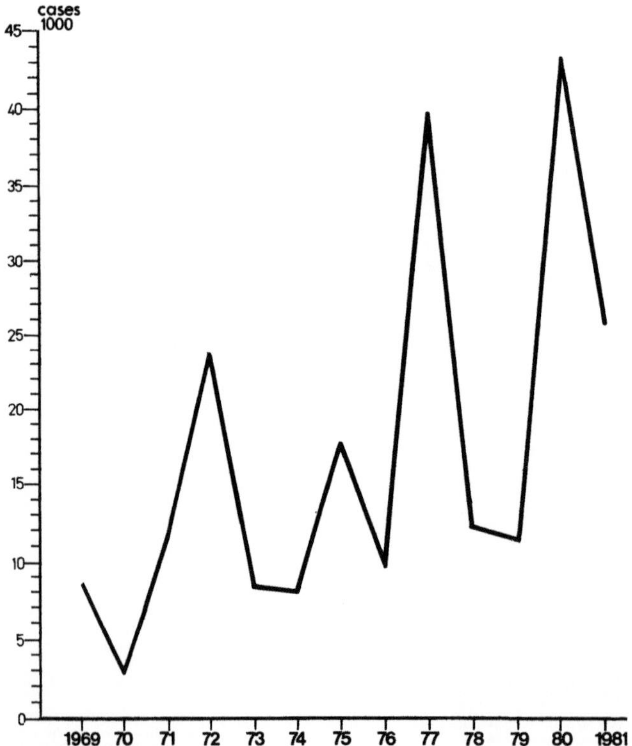

Fig. 10. Dengue haemorrhagic fever in Thailand, 1969–1981

From the very beginning the infection peak had occurred during the summer months and appeared to have a temporal relationship with the onset of the south west monsoon rains.

The situation in 1970, the beginning of the ten year period under investigation, was as follows: DHF had entered almost all of Thailand's provinces, with some provinces being particularly seriously affected. The disease manifested a seasonal dynamic, represented in the rise in the number of cases during the months from June to October, along with a decline during the winter months (Diagram Plate 4). The original two-year rhythm was no longer recognisable. Predictions concerning time and space seemed impossible, apart from the fact that a further spatial spread had to be expected.

4 Study Findings

4.1 Material and Methods

Since 1969 the complete weekly numbers of DHF cases reported by each of the 72 provinces of Thailand have been made available to the Geomedical Research Unit Heidelberg by the Ministry of Public Health in Bangkok. For the study presented here the 10-year period from January, 1970, to December, 1979, was selected. Choropleth maps[3] followed by isarithmic maps[4] with data which had been added at an earlier stage, were produced by computer on the basis of the GEOMAP-Program of Waterloo University in Ontario, Canada, the modified version of which had kindly been made available for use by the Geographical Institute of the University of Heidelberg (Director Prof. Fricke).

Being in the form of weekly records, the data allowed an analysis of the seasonal dynamics for each of the provinces to be carried out in conjunction with the temperature and precipitation data supplied by the Meteorological Department of the Ministry of Communications in Bangkok, so far as weather stations existed. In the event the *Atlas of Thailand*, which had been compiled by Prof. Dr. U. Freitag on behalf of the Royal Thai Survey Department, Bangkok, was also available.

On a visit to Thailand in 1980, the author was able to collect supplementary material as well as to visit hospitals with cases of DHF.

The system of recording is well organized (see Fig. 11). The health officer opens a record on every patient (see Appendix), and passes it on to the local area health office. The data thus collected are collated step-wise, finally reaching the Ministry of Public Health where, together with the original morbidity identification cards, they are differentially processed. Unfortunately, however, the data arriving there are only as good as the quality of their original collection at the local level − as happens everywhere in the world − and at that point there are numerous possibilities for incomplete statistical handling.

To start with, not every sick person is seen by a doctor or at a health centre. In milder cases patients frequently attend the outpatient department of the hospital where notification of cases may or may not be practiced. Nonetheless, it is generally held that in recent years data collection has been carried out with greater care and consistency. Cases admitted to hospital may be assumed to be reported. However, serological tests are only carried out in about 1 in 4 cases. A

---

[3] Choropleth map = shading map, relates a quantity to a certain area.

[4] Isarithm map = continuous distribution of factual data over space (independent of administrative boundaries), represented by lines of equal value obtained by interpolation.

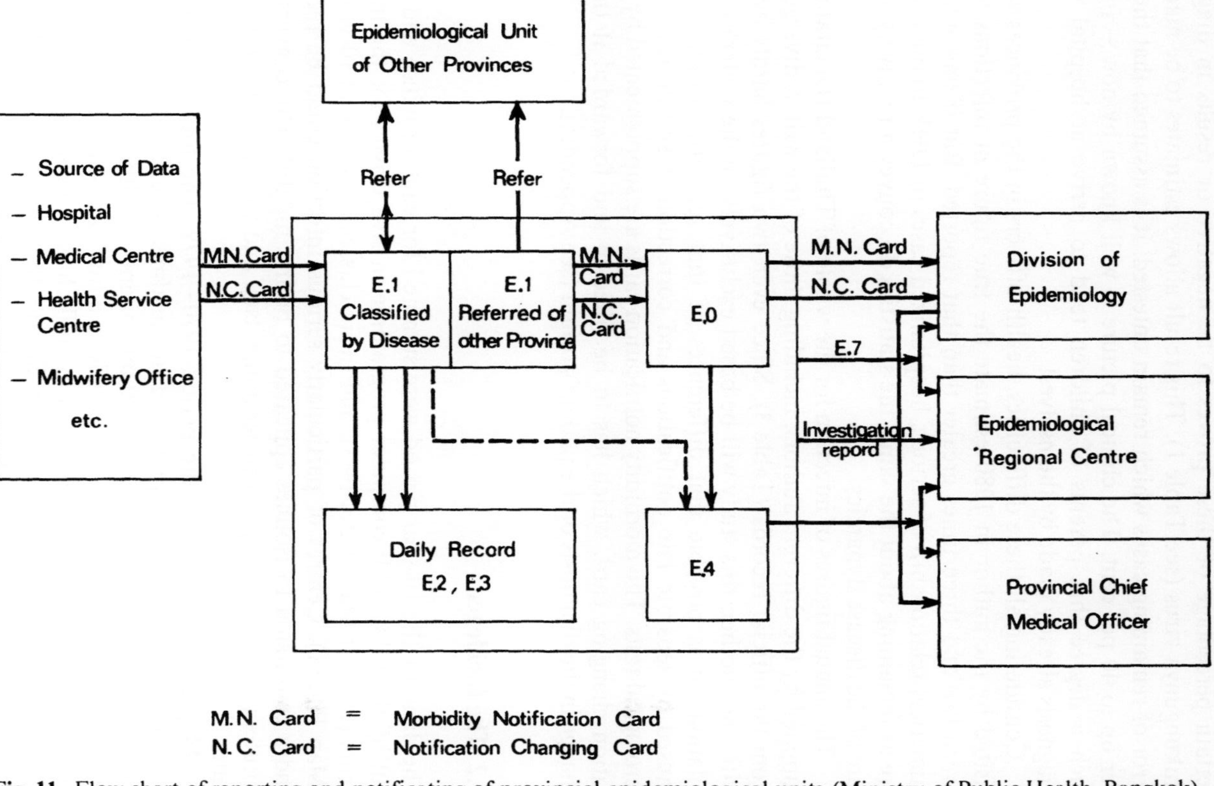

Fig. 11. Flow chart of reporting and notificating of provincial epidemiological units (Ministry of Public Health, Bangkok)

certain percentage of these proves to be negative or results in diagnosis of chikungunya virus (see Table 1). This result allows estimates to be made of the error of remaining cases which remain untested: it is assumed that these number up to 40 per cent. The clinical picture is well known by now – indeed, to such a degree that parents of children tend to arrive at hospital with the diagnosis already made by themselves!

Considering all these difficulties, health officers in the provinces who were visited by the author in 1980 estimate the true figure of infections to be between two and three times greater than that reported. But if one assumes the numerical relationship of serious, hospitalized cases of DHF to the overall figure as remaining about the same, the statistics do convey a relatively good picture of the disease dynamics.

The annual figures of infection for the whole of Thailand (Diagram Plate 4) supplied by the different authors, including those of the writer, diverge slightly from the official records (Table 3). Since even two figures hardly ever agree with one another, this study will be based exclusively on the writer's own compilations. It is possible that differences of that sort arise through mistakes caused by separate late notifications and corrections resulting from negative serological tests. The morbidity notification cards are supplemented by a notification changing card, which has to be filled-in and forwarded if there is a change in the diagnosis or the patient's origin (see Appendix).

4.2 The Incidence

The data for the 10-year period were summed for each province and printed-out by the GEOMAP computer programme in five classes for the individual years (Back of Map Plates 1–3), and in six classes for the total 10-year period (Map Plate 1). Centres of particularly serious infection could be recognised, and a conversion to isolines appeared to be meaningful. The conversion constitutes part of the computer programme itself and was carried out by the computer.

Map Plate 1 represents the period 1970–1979. The total number of cases per 10,000 inhabitants is represented in isarithms. The scale ranges from 0–14 to 101–170 cases of DHF per 10,000 inhabitants over the ten years. Taking the 10-year period as a whole the map reflects a low rate of infection in the mountains of the North and the West, in the hill chains surrounding the Korat Plateau and in the extreme North East. So too, the Thai portion of the Malayan Peninsula is distinctly less affected. The north-eastern and southern Central Plain, however, together with the South East, the centre of the Korat Plateau and the extreme east around Ubon Ratchathani stand out as areas with a large number of people infected with DHF in relation to the numbers of population. An attempt to explain these differences will be made in what follows, in so far as this is possible with the relatively coarse grid of data at provincial level.

First of all attention is directed to the isarithm maps of the ten individual years (1970–1979) which have been derived from the same principle, although they are sub-divided into only five classes, their scale ranging from 0–1 to 301–500 cases of DHF per 100,000 inhabitants.

Throughout the years the main areas of infection represented in Map Plate 1 report a greater or smaller number of cases of DHF as compared with the country's average. In the less seriously affected parts of the country on the other hand, there is a succession of 1−2 years with relatively numerous cases followed by 1−2 years with relatively few cases. However, peak values, are never attained in these areas. This rhythm is not, however, the same throughout the country. On the contrary, each region requires separate consideration in order to be appreciated.

The years 1972, 1975 and 1977 − all of them ones with serious epidemics − were preceded by years during which the pattern of distribution was very similar to that of the map of total numbers (Map Plate 1), even if differences in the degree of infestation were much smaller. The graphs of annual totals for Thailand as a whole (notification of absolute figures) which accompany each of the small maps and specify each month of the corresponding year, show the disease to be virtually at a standstill during the January and February of 1970 and 1971, whilst remaining essentially above 100 cases per month since 1972.

4.3 The Endemic Area

In the *Atlas of Thailand* U. Freitag differentiates four climatic regions (A−D), which are in turn divided into 1 to 5 sub-regions in accordance with precipitation totals (1−5) where 1 indicates the largest and 5 the smallest precipitation amount. Of the 72 provinces of Thailand, 35 are clearly located in one of these climatic regions and were evaluated for this analysis (Table 4). They are located in climatic regions A 1 and A 2, B 2 and B 5, C 1 and C 2 and D 1. In addition provinces in the Northern Region which overlap from B 5 to B 4, and from B 5 to C 3 as a result of their being markedly split-up by river valleys, were also evaluated. This approach seemed acceptable since their climates are fairly similar to each other.

Having thus arrived at groupings of the provinces from the same climatic regions, a curve of the annual mean numbers of notified cases of sickness per 100,000 inhabitants was constructed according to the following formula:

$$M = \frac{DHF_{cl}}{Inh_{cl}} \times 100,000$$

M	= mean monthly value of reported cases
DHF_{cl}	= monthly value of reported cases of all provinces in the climatic region
Inh_{cl}	= total number of inhabitants of all provinces in the climatic region
cl	= climatic region

The mean value was taken from the period 1970-1979. This resulted in 9 graphs of annual means, each of which represents one climatic region. Some climatic regions could not be considered, because the area of no one province is lying entirely within their boundaries. These 9 graphs can in turn be reduced to 3 graph-types, the Trat Province being the sole exception. From north to south the 3 graph-types are arranged as follows (Fig. 12).

Table 4. Grouping of provinces according to climatic regions

Climatic region	Names of provinces	Total No. of inhabitants (1971)
A 1	61 Ranong 62 Phangnga 63 Phuket 64 Krabi 65 Trang 66 Satun	887,451
A 1	49 Trat	94,119
A 2	58 Chumphon 59 Surat Thani 60 Nakhon Si Thammarat 67 Phattalung 68 Songkhla 69 Pattani 70 Yala 71 Narathiwat	3,384,223
B 2	38 Pathum Thani 39 Nonthaburi 40 Krung Thep 41 Thon Buri 46 Chon Buri 47 Rayong	4,372,655
B 5 (+ small areas of B 4)	01 Chiang Rai 02 Mae Hong Son 07 Nan	1,526,501
C 1	18 Nong Khai 19 Udon Thani 20 Sakon Nakhon 21 Nakhon Phanom 72 Yasothon	2,720,429
C 2	37 Ayuthaya 52 Nakhon Pathon 54 Samut Songkhram	1,083,582
D 1	22 Khon Kaen 34 Sing Buri 35 Chai Nat	1,475,540

1. In the humid *Mountain Region* of the extreme N and NW (B 5 and B 4) the peak of the curve remains below 40 cases per 100,000 inhabitants. In winter the disease comes to a complete standstill. So too in the contiguous hill country to the south, and in the relatively humid NE (B 5 and C 3) winter brings a pause, but the graph rises much more steeply here, reaching values far in excess of 100 cases per 100,000 inhabitants in July.

2. The course of the graphs in the drier climates of the *Central Plain and the Korat Plateau* (D 1) looks quite different. Here even the winter months always produce some cases of DHF, and the equally steep rise of the curve in May/June gives to a 'plateau' lasting from July to October. In this instance, monthly figures rise to 90−120 cases per 100,000 inhabitants.

3. The *Southern Peninsula* is situated in the realm of the permanently humid tropics; a central mountain ridge, running north to south, divides the peninsula into a western part with summer rainfall brought along by the SW Monsoon, and an eastern part subject to the winter rains of the NE Monsoon. For all these differences in the annual precipitation regime the summer graphs of DHF infections are identical (A 1 and A 2), resembling that of the northern mountains with a break in winter and a low peak of only some 40 cases per 100,000 inhabitants in July.

In spite of the same climatic influences bearing upon *the Trat Province*, conditions here in the extreme south east of Thailand are evidently different. Infections with DHF are reported here during the winter months as well, and with 270 cases per 100,000 inhabitants, the July peak reaches the highest value in the country as a whole over the 10 year period (province 49, A 1). These obvious differences were the reason for not treating this province together with the Malayan Peninsula, although it is situated in the A 1 climatic region. For this reason the fact will have to be taken into account when evaluating this graph that the population figure of 94,119 is a very small one upon which to base it. The divergence could therefore be relatively large. All the other 8 graphs in Map Plate 2 are based on population figures for 3 to 8 provinces each, which vary in the number of their inhabitants from 981,570 to 4,372,655.

The graphs of the B 2, C 2 and D 1 climatic regions bear a close resemblance to one another. A comparison with temperature and precipitation curves show

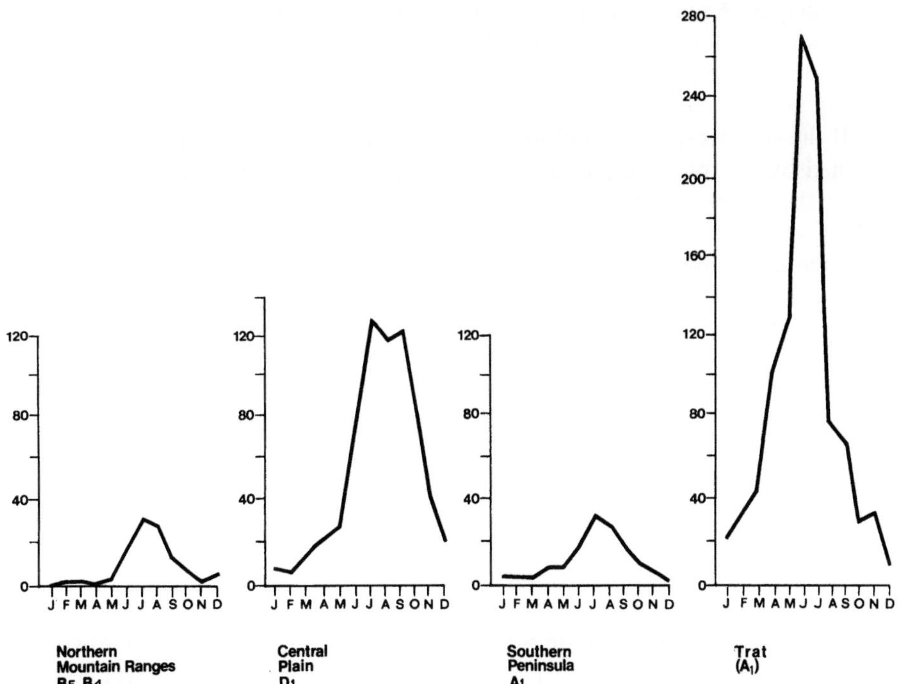

Fig. 12. Seasonality of dengue haemorrhagic fever in 4 selected climatic regions. Cases per 100,000 inhabitants in 10 years

that they are situated in areas which in the course of the year rarely achieve a precipitation surplus over evaporation. On the basis of this observation, the following interpretation is put forward.

In the arid areas of Thailand discussed above (namely B 2, C 2 and D 1) it is common practice to collect water in large earthenware containers for drinking purposes and other general uses (see chapter 2.3). These earthenware vessels have to be large and numerous in order to catch as much as possible of the occasional rain showers. In attempting to enlarge the catchment area, gutters and pipes conduct the rain from the roof down to the vessels so that the entire rooftop becomes a collecting pan (Fig. 6 and 7). For this reason, as well as reasons of convenience, these vessels are placed very close to the house concerned. Additionally, they are hardly ever completely drained. Both these facts combine to create ideal conditions for breeding as well as feeding *Aedes aegypti*. This would explain the increase in the number of DHF infections two months after the onset of the summer monsoon rains, as well as the levelling-off of the curve (D 1) well into October, since the water levels in the vessels keep fluctuating throughout the rainy season, thereby enabling the mosquito eggs deposited above the water mark to be wetted by every subsequent rainfall and to hatch out. This would also serve to explain the absence of any complete disappearance of the disease during the winter months, since the large number of vessels enables a certain number of mosquitoes to continue breeding.

Quite a different situation would exist in the permanently humid south where water storage is not necessary. Admittedly this does not explain the seasonality of occurrence which has also been observed there; on both sides of the Malayan Peninsula it quite obviously depends upon the onset of the SW Monsoon and not on maximal rainfall which would lead one to expect a peak infection on the eastern side in November/December in accordance with the NE Monsoon.

If the comparatively small numbers of cases in the south of Thailand is explained by the more ample precipitation and the resulting lessened storage of water, the reduced number of notifications in the extreme north may be the result of wintery temperatures. For 1 to 3 months a year the monthly averages here remain below 22 °C, a mean temperature which causes *Aedes aegypti* to cease breeding. This results in an overall low level of mosquito population. This may also be the reason for Aiken's inability to record *Aedes aegypti* in Thailand at altitudes over 1,000 m above sea-level (Aiken, 1977).

In contrast to the northern and southern parts of the country, central Thailand and the Korat Plateau could thus be regarded as endemic areas, represented here by a delimiting line in accordance with U. Freitag's map of the climatic regions (Map Plate 2).

4.4 DHF and the Main Transport Routes

The first evidence of a dengue virus in a patient with haemorrhagic fever was adduced in Bangkok in 1958. Throughout South East Asia the ports were the first places in which the disease was to be observed, and in which evidence could be adduced. Very soon, however, the disease was reported from other towns in the interior as well, and this gave rise to the assumption that diffusion took place along the main transport routes. According to McDonald (1956) to so-called mechanical diffusion of aedes eggs — which retain their ability to survive for a long time if dried-out slowly — takes place by means of trains and ships.

For this reason an attempt has been made to reconstruct the diffusion routes in Thailand on the periphery (Text Map 4) by representing the provinces at three different stages of the period with a first sudden rise in numbers of infected persons exceeding 100 cases per year spatially related to the main communication routes.

Apart from the provinces of the South East, which enjoy a very good road link with Bangkok, the provinces affected by 1970 are seen to be situated along the railways, as was to be expected, thus confirming the pertinent conjectures of other authors. For the provinces of the South East transport of *Aedes* eggs by lorries may be considered.

4.5 DHF and the Urban Population

The urban population has increased greatly during the years which saw the rise of DHF in Thailand. In 1960 only 20 towns had more than 20,000 inhabitants, whereas in 1972, the year of the first country-wide epidemic (with 23,560 reported cases of infection), their number had had increased to 31, and another 11 towns had more than 50,000 inhabitants each. These towns are shown in Text Map 5. In this map these provinces are picked out in hatching where DHF infections per 1,000 inhabitants were higher than the national average. Unfortunately there does not seem to be another way of representing the particular rate of infection among the urban population with the relatively coarse data set of a province as the basic unit. But this much may be observed — namely, that DHF occurs more frequently in places which have experienced a substantial increase in their urban population. These are especially the provinces whose capitals passed the 20,000 mark between 1960 and 1972, or grew from 20,000 to more than 50,000 inhabitants. The Malayan Peninsula and the North should not be included in these considerations because of their special climatic circumstances.

If the provinces with growing capitals are affected in excess of others, Surin, Chachaengsao and Suphan Buri would have to expect an increase in infections in the near future — an event already beginning to materialise in Surin since 1978, in fact.

The particular exposure of the urban population results from the demands of *A. aegypti*, which prefers artificial water containers to natural water. Since even the smallest container, such as are found on refuse tips, is sufficient to hold enough rainwater for one batch of mosquito eggs, a town offers prolific possibilities, but increasing numbers of cases have recently been reported from the rural areas as well.

4
Railways and onset
of epidemic spread of
dengue haemorrhagic fever
Trains (all types)
per day
20-40
< 20
First increase of more than 100 cases
of DHF per year by provinces
1970 and bevore
1971 - 1975
1976 - 1979
below 100 cases
0   50   100
Km
GFH

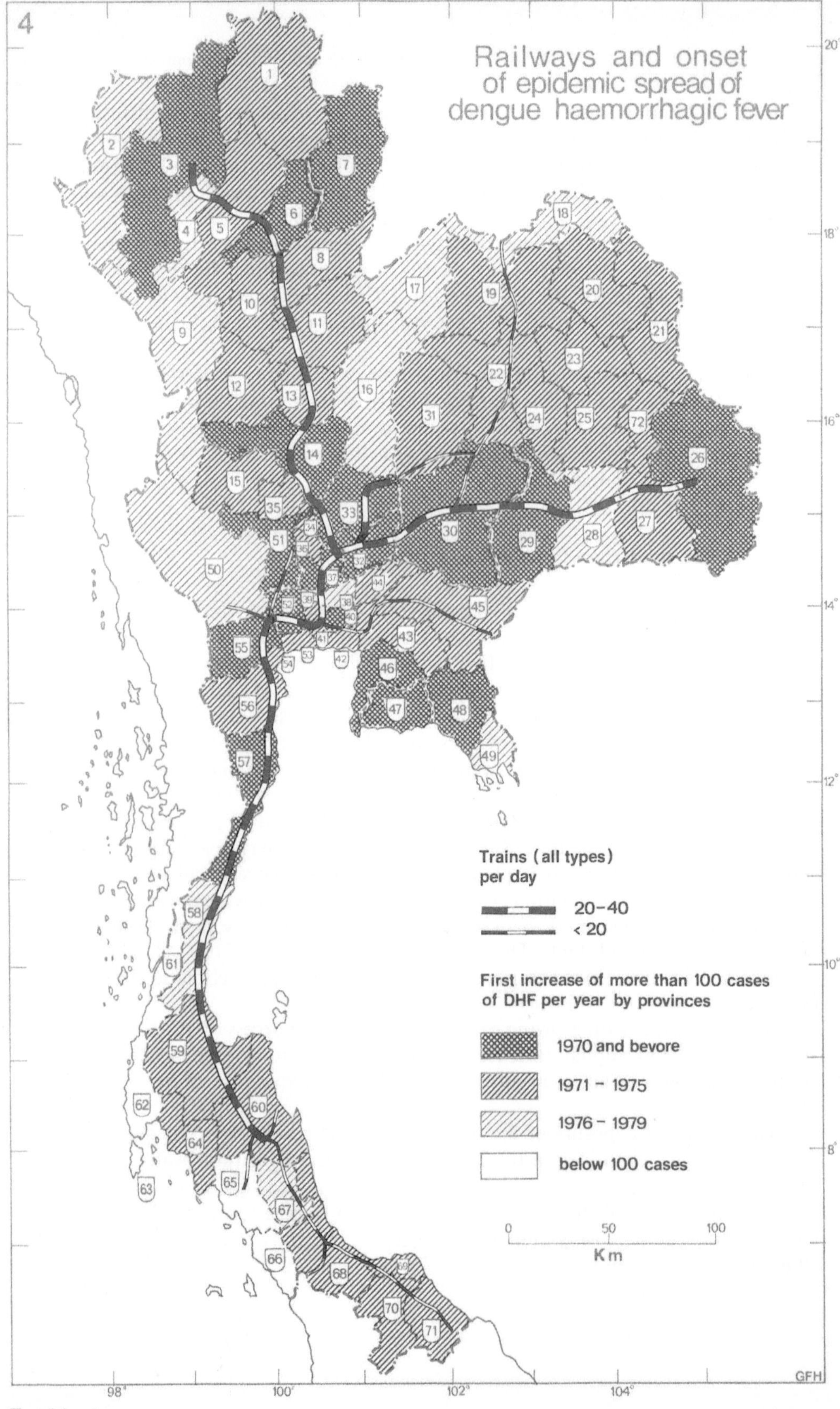

Text Map 4

5
Urban population
and
dengue haemorrhagic fever
DHF per 1 000 inh.
for 10 years
above average
average
below average
Inhabitants
No growth
1960 > 20 000
1972 > 20 000
1960 > 50 000
1972 > 50 000
Rapid growth
1960 < 20 000
1972 > 20 000
1960 < 20 000
1972 > 50 000
1960 > 20 000
1972 > 50 000
GFH

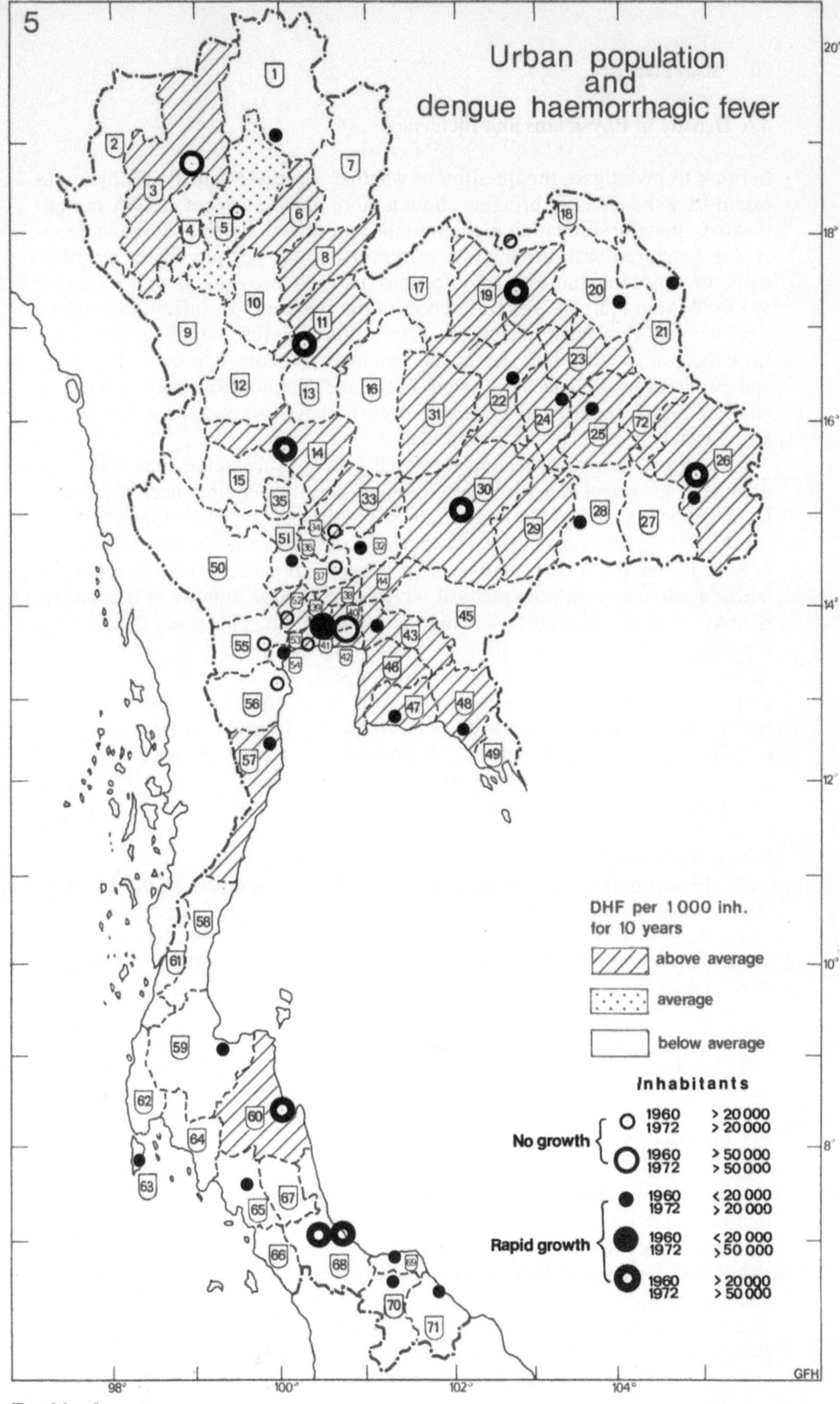

Text Map 5

4.6 Density of Physicians and Incidence

In order to investigate the question of whether a greater density of physicians would have the effect of bringing about a more intense level of activity in notifications, thereby simulating higher numbers of infections, the physician density was compared with the number of reported cases per physician as well as with the absolute numbers of infections in each province over the period 1970–79 (Map Plate 3). The differences in the frequency of infections between this map and Map Plate 1 (Number of infections per 100,000 inhabitants) consist chiefly of the different size of the provinces. Of course, provinces as large and populous as Chiang Mai, Udon Thani and Nakhon Ratchasima have, in absolute terms, reported many cases, even if they do not appear among the most severely affected areas in Map Plate 1.

The errors in data collection may well be very substantial, but it is quite definitely not correlated with the physician density per province. This statement can be verified by the Map Plate 3. The basis is given by the number of inhabitants per physician. The red hatching indicates the number of infected persons in relation to the number of inhabitants. If there were a direct correlation, a province with poor medical services, i.e. a large number of inhabitants per physician, would report a low number of infections. This is not the case. On the contrary the whole spectrum of possibilities is there, from the medically speaking very well supplied area around Bangkok with few cases per physician despite the high numbers of infections with DHF, to the medically still well provided Chantaburi in the south east where, in an area having a relatively high number of cases, each doctor also reports many cases; from Pichit, which has only three physicians but many cases reported by each one of them in an area having a low absolute number of infections, to the medically equally poorly served Nong Khai reporting few cases per physician in an area of low overall total notifications.

If the assumption that many doctors equal high numbers of notifications and the reverse, that few doctors equal low numbers of notifications, were correct, the number of inhabitants per physician would be the negative of the absolute numbers of infections, and the number of infected persons per physician (red symbol) the same throughout Thailand.

Thanks to these considerations we assume that the number of notifications per province – at least in their relation to each other – corresponds with the facts, and that the statements made on the maps are correct.

4.7 Seasonality

There has been repeated mention of the correlation between the rise in the number of DHF notifications and the onset of the south west monsoon. In order to examine this inter-relationship the precipitation curves of existing weather stations for the period 1970–79 have been represented in conjunction with the relevant numbers of DHF infections, also in the form of graphs (Diagram Plate 4). The inter-relationship between the onset of the south west monsoonal rains and the rise in the frequency of infections was confirmed in all the provinces in so far as the latter followed the former at an interval of one month. This interval confirms the following calculation: the eggs of *Aedes*, deposited in vessels, are wetted by rising water-levels and larvae develop within a few hours. About one week later the adults hatch and are immediately capable of biting (and potential infection); after 4 to 5 days they deposit their eggs, the development of which is set in train by the next rainfall. Thus the mosquito population grows. After the second depositing of eggs the proportion of infected females has increased so much that the rate of transmission reaches a relatively high level, and the epidemic breaks out. This dependency is demonstrated in the Diagram Plate which shows the graphs for precipitation and for the number of infections in four provinces from different climatic regions.

The seasonal dynamic of the Songkhla Province presents a problem which has already been discussed elsewhere (WHO *Epidemiological Record* 8, 1969 and Aiken, 1977), namely the question of whether there is a seasonal peak in the biting activity of *A. aegypti*, that is independent of precipitation or possibly favoured by it. Songkhla receives the greater amount of its precipitation in the winter months at the time of the north east monsoons; the peak of infections nonetheless occurs during the time of the summer (south-west) monsoon as everywhere else in Thailand, although it turns out to be rather weaker in Songkhla, as the precipitation falls on the hills of the west coast of the Malayan Peninsula, and Songkhla is situated on the east coast. This would imply postulating a seasonal rhythm in the behaviour of *A. aegypti*, with a rise in the biting activity during the months of May to August, which is subsequently varied by the prevailing local precipitation conditions.

In the north of Thailand wintry temperatures constitute an additional rhythmic factor. Monthly mean temperatures below 22 °C suggest temporary, and especially nocturnal, drops to much lower values. According to Aiken (1977) temperature influences the development of larvae, the frequency of bites and the duration of life of *A. aegypti*. Larval development ceases at 15−20 °C, and below 18 °C the adult mosquito does not bite any more. It is on that account that the 20 °C isotherm has been found empirically to present the limit of *Aedes aegypti's* distribution. A. W. A. Brown delimits the zone of permanent habitation by the 10 °C July isotherm in the Southern hemisphere; and in the northern hemisphere takes the 10 °C January isotherm. As a high population density of mosquitoes is required to spread epidemics, diseases transmitted by *A. aegypti* are likely to inhabit an area smaller than that delimited by the 10 °C annual isotherm.

5 Conclusions

It has proved possible to demonstrate that the figures for DHF notifications, which are unevenly distributed throughout the country, are independent of physician density. This is to challenge the argument that improved medical services would result in higher numbers of notifications, whereas poor medical services would leave doctors little time or interest for filling in the detailed notification papers. Notification is not carried out by the doctor himself in Thailand, but as a rule by a health worker at the basic level, or, as the case may be, by a health official at the local health service office who visits hospitals at regular intervals. Although a largish number, or even the majority, of the less serious cases that only attend the outpatients department, are slipping through the statistical net, it can be assumed that the disease dynamic is nonetheless represented by the cases that are admitted to hospital. These presuppositions alone justify further statements. On the other hand any sophisticated statistical procedures were avoided.

Whereas the physical environment − especially the climate − delimits the distribution pattern of an arthropode vector and an infectious agent, it is on the other hand the socio-economic development and the socio-cultural behaviour of a people that is also responsible for the outbreak of an epidemic.

Since, in the first time, *A. aegypti* has used the main transport routes, especially the railway lines, for its diffusion, DHF appears to have followed the same paths into Thailand, too. In any case the provinces which were first affected are situated along the few major lines of rail. The further diffusion does not appear to follow any rules save for the fact that the most peripheral provinces in the south and north were the last to be reached.

However, it is very well recognized that there is a preference for urban centres which have increased greatly during the years since the disease first occurred. Not only do they present the highest absolute figures of DHF, as might be expected, but they also present the highest incidence in relation to the population totals of the province. Favourable conditions for *A. aegypti* are incidental to the rapid growth of settlements in so far as water supplies and refuse removal are usually unable to keep abreast of requirements. The consequence, especially in the arid parts of the country, is a marked tendency to store water and to pile up refuse of all sorts, including cans, car tyres and plastic articles. These man-made vessels are the breeding places for *A. aegypti*, as the female deposits its eggs on the inner walls of such vessels. Thanks to this pronounced link with man and its preference for human blood as its meals, *A. aegypti* has a higher degree of infection with dengue viruses than that of the authochtonous species *A. albopictus*. It would be worthwhile noting the number of containers per house throughout Thailand which could be regarded as potential breeding places for *A. aegypti*. Regional differences might be found which correlate with the distribution of DHF.

During the first decade DHF displayed a 2-year rhythm, i.e. a year of fewer infections occurred between two markedly epidemic years. This rhythm has not been observed since 1968 (see Fig. 10), for it is not a matter of one virus affecting a population that has become well immunized by each preceding epidemic year, but of four serotypes without cross-immunity. So far none of these serotypes has been found to be solely responsible for the DHF. Even the order of secondary infections does not reveal any regularity. Only the interval between primary and secondary infection has been considered as having a causal effect. Amongst others this fact could be regarded as an explanation of the susceptibility of children to DHF. With adults the primary infection tends to have occurred a long term earlier, as dengue is widely distributed in Thailand, and antibodies have been acquired by almost every adult during childhood.

At present the only regularity of the return of the epidemic years might be seen in the similarity of the distribution pattern of the preceding year with the map of total numbers for the 10-year period under review, which would thus present a kind of "normal state". But since this has so far only been observed on three occasions, further developments remain to be expected.

Apart from the different number of cases in individual years DHF in Thailand occurs with a marked seasonal frequency during the summer months. The peaks of the graphs vary greatly from May to July, but remain fairly constant each year as far as the individual provinces are concerned. Two facts require discussion here: the rise in the curve, and the winter pause.

In all the provinces the rise in the curves takes place about 1 to 2 months after the onset of the rains. This would appear to prove an inter-relationship were there not some facts suggesting the possibility that this temporal sequence could be an adaptation by the mosquito population to the climatic conditions, so that *A. aegypti's* most active phase or readiness to bite coincides with the season most favourable for breeding.

Halstead counted five earthenware jars per household in Bangkok and a house index[5] of nearly 100 throughout the year. This would point to the mosquito population remaining constant throughout the year. In Malaysia the so-called ant-traps beneath the legs of furniture or similar articles play an important role. Together with the earthenware jars they account for 51.7 per cent of the breeding places (Cheong, 1967). Although the water in these traps is topped-up regularly and larvae are present, Malaysia also experiences a seasonal dynamic in DHF.

This study also detected an indication in the fact that on the eastern side of the Malayan Peninsula the peak of DHF infections occurs in the wake of the lesser rains of the south west monsoon, while the north east monsoon, with its much more prolific rainfall, is not followed by a second peak of infections.

Another point concerns the break in winter in the north, as well as in the south of Thailand. Its cause may well be different in these two areas. Low temperatures, such as those occurring in the north during some of the winter

---

[5] House index = percentage of houses positive for the species

months, are detrimental to the development of larvae, the frequency of bites and the duration of the life of *A. aegypti*, so that it must be assumed that the northern limit of *A. aegypti*, and thus of DHF, has been reached here. However, consideration must be given to the totally unknown factor of the near complete absence of contact by the mountain peoples of these provinces with the Thais who live in the valleys, and of their rare visits to hospitals. On the other hand, taking into consideration the ecological requirements of *A. aegypti*, which were treated above, DHF does not seem very likely to occur among the mountain peoples.

The winter pause in southern Thailand is to be viewed in a different way. Here temperatures remain high throughout the year and all months are humid. The question arises whether DHF has reached its maximal extent at all in these provinces, or rather whether the course of the graph under identical climatic conditions in the Trat Province in the south east of Thailand (see Map Plate 2) is not representative for the final state of the increase. In Trat the highest values of the country in relation to the population are reached, and there is no break in winter. A factor that cannot be evaluated in this context is the refugee-problem in Trat. Refugee camps can give rise to all sorts of diseases.

Halstead (1969) noted that in the period 1962−64, DHF was absent from all the provinces outside Bangkok during the winter months. This is no longer so, and may be the consequence of the expansion. If that is the case, a considerable increase in DHF might have to be expected in southern Thailand in years to come.

An attempt at a prognosis will be tried here, although it is, of course, a risky enterprise bearing in mind the difficulty of obtaining data mentioned earlier. The rising totals of the peak years (more than 43,000 cases were reported in 1980) suggest a further increase, but may be the outcome of stricter notification. The reasons mentioned above, however, permit the writer to incline to the view that the maximal diffusion has not yet been reached in the south and that expanding towns like Surin, Chachaensao or Suphan Buri, too, will have to expect a further increase. In the north and north east the limit of spread has probably been reached on climatic grounds.

In the 10 computer maps (back of Map Plates 1−3) showing the annual distribution for the individual years 1970−1979, the same areas of maximum infection stand out time and time again. It must be assumed that the number of cases per inhabitants unit will remain high here in years to come. The reasons for this are still unknown. Extensive field studies on the possibility of delimiting an endemic area will be required to this end.

Acknowledgement

This book is the result of a long period of effort, support and patience from many sides.

When Prof. em. Dr. med. H. J. Jusatz, Geomedical Research Unit of the Heidelberg Academy of Sciences, invited the author for working on the subject, the DHF-data-set meant nothing more than a list of about 50,000 figures to her. But these figures gained life by his scientific guidance and by providing me the occasion to visit the country and its health services. So, to Prof. Dr. H. J. Jusatz, as the initiator of this study, the author is deeply indebted. His co-workers, Mrs. M. Albrecht and Mr. H. Sauer, patiently typed and re-typed, designed and re-designed the outcomes what is very much acknowledged.

Prof. Dr. Dr. Ouay Ketusinh, Bangkok, as a good friend of Prof. Dr. H. J. Jusatz, took the burden to guide me through the country of Thailand and opened with his influence all the doors to universities, ministries, hospitals and health offices. My warmest gratitude is for him who, apart from the scientific support, allowed me also some insight in Thai way of life.

Without the statistics from the Ministry of Public Health in Bangkok, which continued to arrive with unfailing regularity for more than a decade, this study could not have been carried out at all. My thanks are due to its staff, and especially to Dr. Boonthai who found time for personal discussion as well as providing a glimpse into the work of the statistical development by the ministry.

I wish to thank the Department of Meteorology in Bangkok and Professor Dr. M. Domrös, Institute of Geography, University Mainz for climate data, and Prof. Dr. U. Freitag, Institute of Anthropogeography, Geography and Cartography, Free University Berlin for his readiness in presenting me with some proofs from the Atlas of Thailand and for his cartographic advise. Prof. Dr. W. Fricke, Geographical Institute of Heidelberg University very kindly made the GEOMAP-Program available to me for producing computer maps. The use of the computer was financially supported by the Deutsche Forschungsgemeinschaft, Bonn, what is greatly acknowledged.

I am very grateful to Dr. J. A. Hellen, Newcastle upon Tyne and Mrs. J. F. Hellen for the translation into English as well as to the many who kindly supported my research during my stay in Thailand.

Miss B. Timmermann und Miss E. Mechelke are to be thanked for their hard work in the processing of large quantities of data.

Finally, the author thanks the "Kartographisches Atelier und Offsetdruckerei Henning Wocke" in Karlsruhe for the careful printing of the maps and the Springer Verlag in Heidelberg for the good lay-out of the text, diagrams and photographs.

References

Aiken SR, Leigh CH (1978) Dengue haemorrhagic Fever in Southeast Asia. Trans Inst Brit Geogr 3, 4:476–497

Aiken SR, Frost DB, Leigh CH (1980) Dengue Haemorrhagic Fever and rainfall in peninsular Malaysia: some suggested relationships. Soc Sci Med 14 D 3:307–316

Avril W (1972) Dengue Hämorrhagisches Fieber in Südasien. Diss Reihe des Südasien-Instituts der Universität Heidelberg Bd 14

Atlas of Thailand (1977) Royal Thai Survey Department

Brown AWA (1977) Yellow fever, dengue and dengue haemorrhagic fever. In: Howe GM (ed) A world geography of human diseases. Academic Press, London New York San Francisco, p 271–317

Chan YC, Chan KC, Ho BC (1971) *Aedes aegypti* and *Aedes albopictus* in Singapur. Bull WHO 44:617–657

Cheong WH (1967) Preferred *Aedes aegypti* larval habitats in urban areas. Bull WHO 36:586–589

Downs WG (1981) A new look at yellow fever and malaria; Soper lecture 7 Nov 1980. Am J Trop Med Hyg 30:516–522

Denner W (1972) Zur Wirtschaftsgeographie Thailands. Ztschr Wirtschaftsgeogr H 1:1–7

Denner W (1976) Zur Wirtschaftsgeographie Thailands. Ztschr Wirtschaftsgeogr H 4:108–116

Fraser HS, Wilson WA, Thomas EJ, et al. (1978) Dengue shock syndrome in Jamaica. Br Med J 1:893–894

Freitag U (1980) Concept, Design and Production of the new "Atlas of Thailand". Geo-Journal 4:76–79

Halstead SB, Yamarat C (1965) Recent epidemics of haemorrhagic fever in Thailand. Observations related to pathogenesis of a "new" dengue disease. Am J Publ Health 55:1386–1395

Halstead SB (1966) Epidemiological studies of Thai haemorrhagic fever 1962–1964. Bull WHO 35:80–81

Halstead SB et al. (1969) Dengue and chikungunya virus infection in men in Thailand, 1962–64. II. Am J Trop Med Hyg 18:972–983; III. 984–996; IV. 997–1021; 1022–1034

Halstead SB (1980) Dengue haemorrhagic fever – a public health problem and a field for research. Bull WHO 58, 1:1–21

Halstead SB (1981) The pathogenesis of dengue. Molecular Epidemiology in infectious disease. Am J Epid 114:632–648

Halstead SB (1982) WHO fights dengue haemorrhagic fever. WHO Chron 38, 2:65–67

Hammon W McD, Rudnick A, Sather GE (1960) Viruses associated with epidemic hemorrhagic fevers of the Philippines and Thailand. Science 131:1102

Howe GM (ed) (1977) A world geography of human diseases. Academic Press, London New York San Francisco

Jatanasen S (1966) Occurrence of haemorrhagic fever in Thailand 1958–64. Bull WHO 35:79–80

Jusatz HJ (1972) Gegenwärtige Verbreitung des Dengue Hämorrhagischen Fiebers in Südasien. Med Klinik 5:152–156

Jusatz HJ (1975) The present distribution of dengue haemorrhagic fever in South Asia. Applied Sciences and Development 6:119–126

Knudsen AB (1977) The silent jungle transmission of dengue virus and its tenable relationship to dengue in Malaysia. The Malayan Nature J 31, 1:41–48 (1977)

Landsberg R, Meyers WR, Davis R et al. (1980) Dengue-Texas. Morbidity and Mortality Weekly Report 29:451

Lopez-Correa RH, Cline BL, Ramirez-Ronda C, et al. (1978) Dengue fever with hemorrhagic manifestations: a report of three cases from Puerto Rico. Am J Trop Med Hyg 27:1216–1224

Maas W (1963) Hinterindien. In: Die große illustrierte Länderkunde. Bertelsmann Lexikon Institut, Gütersloh 1:1186–1262

Maede M (1976) A new disease in Southeast Asia: mans creation of dengue haemorrhagic fever. Pacific viewpoint 17, 2:133–146

Melnick JL (1980) Taxonomy of Viruses, 1980. Prog med Virol (Basel) 26:214–232

Morbidity and Mortality Weekly Report (1980) Dengue – Texas. 29:407–408

Nimmannitya S, Halstead SB et al. (1969) Dengue and chikungunya virus infection in man in Thailand, 1962–64. I. Observations on hospitalized patients with Hemorrhagic fever. Am J Trop Med Hyg 18:954–971

Pant DB, Jatanasen S, Yasund M (1973) Prevalence of *Aedes aegypti* and *Aedes albopictus* and observations on the ecology of DHF in several areas in Thailand. Southeast Asian J Trop Med Publ Health 4:113–121

Rodenwaldt E, Jusatz HJ (eds) (1952–1961) Welt-Seuchen-Atlas – World Atlas of Epidemic Diseases. Falk Hamburg, Bd I–III

Rudnik A, Hammon W (1961) Entomological aspects of Thai haemorrhagic fever epidemics in Bangkok, the Philippines and Singapore 1956–61. Proc Thai Haemorrh. Fever Symposium Seato Bangkok, Med Res Monograph 2:24–29

Rudnik A (1967) *Aedes aegypti* and haemorrhagic fever. Bull WHO 36:528–532

Scanlon JE (1966) The distribution of *Aedes aegypti* in Thailand. Bull WHO 35:81–82

Simpson DIH (1978) Dengue haemorrhagic fever – a public health problem and a field for research. Bull WHO 56, 6:819–832

Smith CEG (1956) The history of dengue in tropical Asia and its probable relationships to the mosquito *Aedes aegypti*. J Trop Med Hyg 59:243–251

Surtees G (1971) Urbanization and the epidemiology of mosquito-borne disease. Abstr Hyg 46, 2:121–134

Sternstein L (1976) Thailand. The environment of modernisation. McGraw-Hill, Sidney

Ulmann E (1961) The Geographical Distribution of Dengue up to 1957. In: Rodenwaldt E, Jusatz HJ (eds) Welt-Seuchen-Atlas – World Atlas of Epidemic Diseases vol III. Falk, Hamburg, III/51–54

WHO (1980) Guide for diagnosis, treatment and control of dengue haemorrhagic fever. 2nd edn. Geneva

WHO (1981) Wkly epid rec 36:237–238

WHO (1981) Wkly epid rec 36:379

WHO (1982) Wkly epid rec 37:176

Appendix

Morbidity Notification Card

O Smallpox	Dysentery:	O Influenza
O Cholera	O Bacillary	Hepatitis:
O Plague	O Amoebic	O Infectious, A.
O Yellow Fever	O Unspecified	O Serum, B.
O Meningococcal Meningitis	O Amoebiasis (other organs)	O Unspecified
O Scrub Typhus	O Poliomyelitis	O Infectious Yaws
O Dengue Haemorrhagic Fever	Encephalitis:	O Malaria
O Diphtheria	O Japanese B.	O Leprosy
O Pertussis	O Post Infection	Tuberculosis:
O Tetanus	O Post Vaccination	O Pulmonary
O Acute Diarrhoea	O Unspecified	O Other Systems
O Food Poisoning	O Rabies	O Phyrexia of Unknown Origin
O Enteric Fever	O Measles	O Conjunctivitis (epidemica)
O Typhoid Fever	O Rubella	O Accidental Poisoning by
O Parathyphoid Fever	O Chickenpox	Insecticide
		O Occupational disease

Card number . . . . *Hospital number* . . . .

Patient's name . . . .

Parent's name (for child) . . . .

Date of birth . . . . Age . . . . . . Year . . . . . . Month . . . . . . Day . . . . . . Sex   O Male
Nationality   O Thai   O Chinese   O Others   O Female
Religion   O Buddhism   O Islam   O Christian   O Others
Marital Status   O Single   O Married   O Separated   O Divorced   O Widow
Occupation . . . .

Patient's address

House No. . . . . . . Lane . . . . Street . . . . Hamlet number . . . . . .

Name of Hamlet . . . . Sub-district . . . . District . . . .

Province . . . .

Municipality   O Inside   O Outside

Date of onset . . . . Date of admission . . . .
Hospitalization   O Hospital
O In patient   O Health centre
O Out patient   O Private clinic
                        O Others

Patient's condition
O Improved   O Recovered   O Escaped   O Dead
O Transfer to   O Others

Date of death . . . .

Place of death . . . .

Reporter's name . . . .

Position . . . .

Date . . . .

Office . . . .")

Notification Changing Card

Change or add data as marked below:

O Disease	O Patient's condition
O Patient's name	O Address while contact disease
O Age	O Date of onset or admission
O Laboratory finding	O Others (i. e. sex, nationality, religion, marital status, occupation hospitalization)

Personal data
Patient's name ....Date of birth ..../......../......
Hospital number ....E.O. card number ....

Disease
First notification ....
Change to ....

Age	O years	*Sex*	O male		*Nationality*	O Thai
	O months		O female			O Chinese
	O days					O ....
Religion	O Buddhist	O Islam	O Christ	O ....
Marital Status	O Single	O Married	O Divorced	O separated	O Widow

Occupation ....

Type of work ....

Patient's address

House number ....Lane ....Street ....

Hamlet name ....Hamlet number ....Sub-district ....

District ....Province ....

Municipality   O Inside

                        O Outside

In case of occupational disease please indicate place of work

Office ....

Address ....

Period of working ....Days ....Month ......Years .....

Date of onset ....*Date of admission* ....

Hospitalization
O hospiatal	O clinic	O home
O inpatient	O health centre	O others
O out patients	O Midwiferey centre	

Patient's condition
O Improved   O Recovered   O Escaped   O Dead   O Unknown   O Others

O Transfer to ....

　Place of death ....

　Date of death ....

Laboratory finding
Diagnosis changed by   O Clinical finding
                                       O Laboratory finding

Laboratory method   O Smear   O Culture   O Serology

Requested on ....

Reported on ....

Result ....

Reporter's name ....

Position ....

Date of reporting ....

Office ....

Province ....

Source: Division of Epidemiology

J. C. Frauenthal

Mathematical Modeling in Epidemiology

Universitext
1980. IX, 118 pages
DM 26,-. ISBN 3-540-10328-7

W. R. Hess, P. G. Howell, D. W. Verwoerd

African Swine Fever Virus. Bluetongue Virus

1971. 5 figures. IV, 74 pages. (Virology Monographs, Volume 9)
Cloth DM 29,-. ISBN 3-211-81006-4

E. Hinz

Schistosoma intercalatum-Infektionen in Afrika Saisonkrankheiten in Nigeria

Beiträge zur Geomedizin der Tropen
1980. 1 Kartenblatt, 8 Abbildungen, 2 Tabellen. 69 Seiten.
(Sitzungsberichte der Heidelberger Akademie der Wissenschaften,
Mathematisch-naturwissenschaftliche Klasse. 1980, 2)
DM 42,-. ISBN 3-540-10160-8

D. L. Ingram, L. E. Mount

Man and Animals in Hot Environments

1975. 84 figures, 14 tables. XI, 185 pages. (Topics in Environmental
Physiology and Medicine). Cloth DM 84,-. ISBN 3-540-06865-1

M. Katz, D. D. Despommier, R. W. Gwadz

Parasitic Diseases

1982. 346 figures (including 33 parasite life cycle drawings and 4
color plates). XII, 264 pages. Cloth DM 96,-. ISBN 3-540-90689-4

B. M. Thimm

Brucellosis

Distribution in Man, Domestic and Wild Animals
1982. With 3 coloured map plates of Europe, Africa and America
and 2 figures. XI, 55 pages. (Sitzungsberichte der Heidelberger Akademie der Wissenschaften, Mathematisch-naturwissenschaftliche
Klasse. 1982, Supplement). Cloth DM 45,-. ISBN 3-540-11232-4

R. A. Wever

The Circadian System of Man

Results of Experiments Under Temporal Isolation
1979. 181 figures, 11 tables. XI, 276 pages. (Topics in Environmental
Physiology and Medicine)
Cloth DM 118,-. ISBN 3-540-90338-0

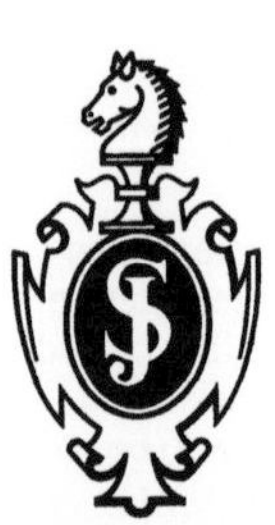

Springer-Verlag
Berlin
Heidelberg
New York
Tokyo

1

DENGUE HAEMORRHAGIC FEVER
IN
THAILAND
1970 – 1979

DENGUE HÄMORRHAGISCHES FIEBER
IN
THAILAND
1970 – 1979

**TOTAL NUMBER OF CASES
PER 10000 INHABITANTS
IN 10 YEARS
(based on Computer Mapping)**

**GESAMTZAHL DER FÄLLE
PRO 10000 EINWOHNER
IN 10 JAHREN
(auf der Grundlage von
Computer-Karten)**

HELLA WELLMER

Cartographic representation:
Geomedical Research Unit
Geomedizinische Forschungsstelle
Helmut J. Jusatz

1. Chiang Rai
2. Mae Hong Son
3. Chiang Mai
4. Lamphun
5. Lampang
6. Phrae
7. Nan
8. Uttaradit
9. Tak
10. Sukhothai
11. Phitsanulok
12. Kamphaeng Phet
13. Phichit
14. Nakhon Sawan
15. Uthai Thani
16. Phetchabun
17. Loei
18. Nong Khai
19. Udon Thani
20. Sakon Nakhon
21. Nakhon Phanom
22. Khon Kaen
23. Kalasin
24. Maha Sarakham
25. Roi Et
26. Ubon Ratchathani

DENGUE HAEMORRHAGIC FEVER
IN THAILAND
1970 – 1974

(based on Computer Mapping)

DENGUE HÄMORRHAGISCHES FIEBER
IN THAILAND
1970 – 1974

(auf der Grundlage von Computer-Karten)

LEGEND / LEGENDE

Incidence per 100 000 inhabitants:
Gemeldete Fälle pro 100 000 Einwohner:

Monthly data
Monatliche Angaben

0– 1

2– 10

11–100

101–300

301–500

Isarithm
Isarithmen

Capital of a Province
Hauptstadt einer Provinz

DENGUE HAEMORRHAGIC FEVER
IN
THAILAND
1970–1979

DENGUE HÄMORRHAGISCHES FIEBER
IN
THAILAND
1970–1979

CLIMATIC REGIONS AND ENDEMIC AREA
KLIMAREGIONEN UND ENDEMIEGEBIET

HELLA WELLMER

Cartographic representation:
Geomedical Research Unit
Geomedizinische Forschungsstelle
Helmut J. Jusatz

1. Chiang Rai
2. Mae Hong Son
3. Chiang Mai
4. Lamphun
5. Lampang
6. Phrae
7. Nan
8. Uttaradit
9. Tak
10. Sukhothai
11. Phitsanulok
12. Kamphaeng Phet
13. Phichit
14. Nakhon Sawan
15. Uthai Thani
16. Phetchabun
17. Loei
18. Nong Khai
19. Udon Thani
20. Sakon Nakhon
21. Nakhon Phanom
22. Khon Kaen
23. Kalasin

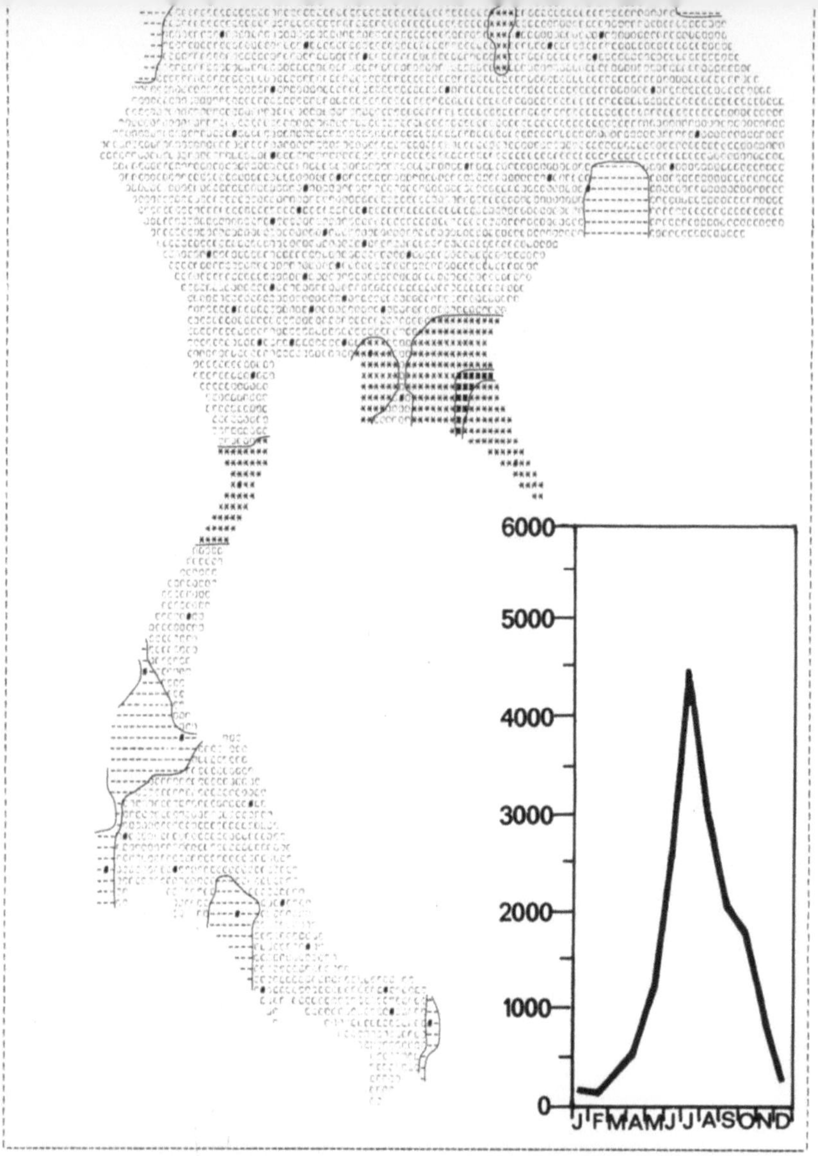

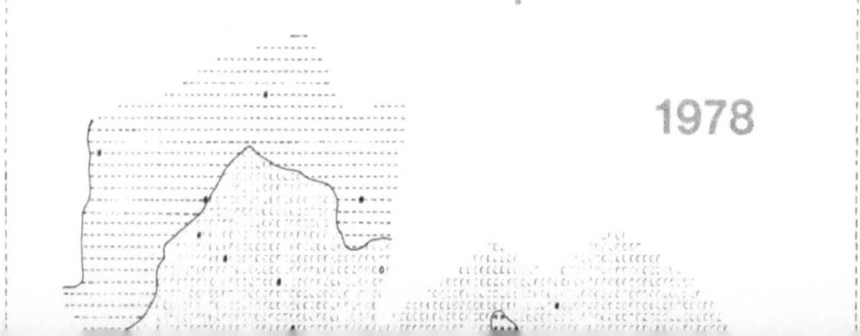

6000
5000
4000
3000
2000
1000
0
J F M A M J J A S O N D
1978

3

DENGUE HAEMORRHAGIC FEVER AND MEDICAL PROVISION IN THAILAND 1970–1979

(based on Computer Mapping)

DENGUE HÄMORRHAGISCHES FIEBER UND ÄRZTLICHE VERSORGUNG IN THAILAND 1970–1979

(auf der Grundlage von Computer-Karten)

HELLA WELLMER

Cartographic representation:
Geomedical Research Unit
Geomedizinische Forschungsstelle
Helmut J. Jusatz

LEGEND / LEGENDE

1. Chiang Rai	39. Nonthaburi
2. Mae Hong Son	40. Phra Nakhon =
3. Chiang Mai	Krung Thep = Bangkok *
4. Lamphun	41. Thon Buri *
5. Lampang	42. Samut Prakan
6. Phrae	43. Chachoengsao
7. Nan	44. Nakhon Nayok
8. Uttaradit	45. Prachin Buri
9. Tak	46. Chon Buri
10. Sukhothai	47. Rayong
11. Phitsanulok	48. Chanthaburi
12. Kanphaeng Phet	49. Trat
13. Phichit	50. Kanchanaburi
14. Nakhon Sawan	51. Suphan Buri
15. Uthai Thani	52. Nakhon Pathom
16. Phetchabun	53. Samut Sakhon
17. Loei	54. Samut Songkhram
18. Nong Khai	55. Ratchaburi
19. Udon Thani	56. Phetchaburi
20. Sakon Nakhon	57. Prachuap Khiri Khan
21. Nakhon Phanom	58. Chum Phon
22. Khon Kaen	59. Surat Thani
23. Kalasin	60. Nakhon Si Thammarat
24. Maha Sarakham	61. Ranong
25. Roi Et	62. Phang-nga
26. Ubon Ratchathani	63. Phuket
27. Si Sa Ket	64. Krabi
28. Surin	65. Trang
29. Burinam	66. Satun
30. Nakhon Ratchasima	67. Phatthalung
31. Chaiyaphum	68. Songkhla
32. Saraburi	69. Pattani
33. Lop Buri	70. Yala
34. Sing Buri	71. Narathiwat
35. Chai Nat	72. Yasothon
36. Ang Thong	

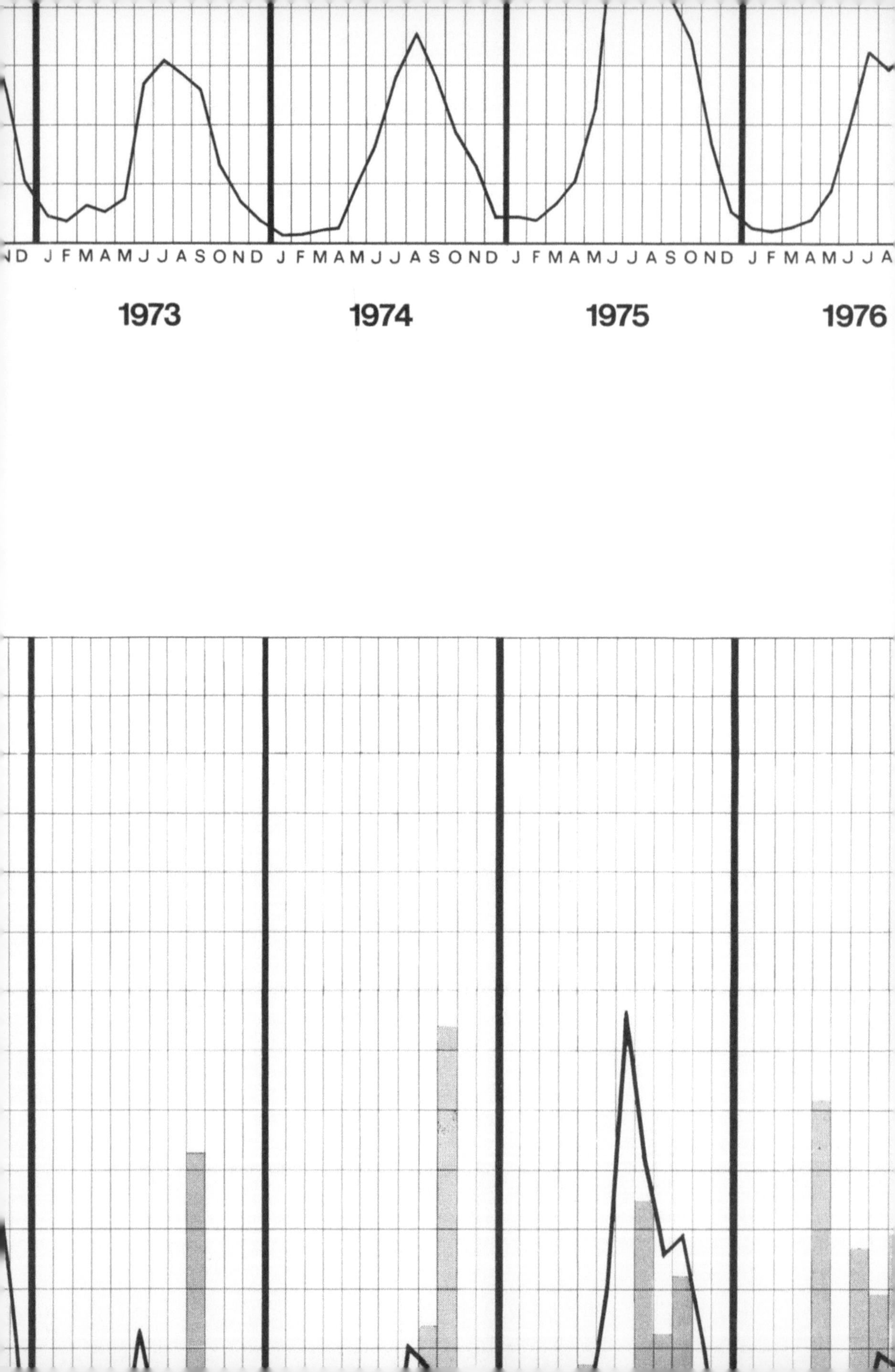

ND J F M A M J J A S O N D J F M A M J J A S O N D J F M A M J J A S O N D J F M A M J J A
1973
1974
1975
1976

INCIDENCE OF DENGUE HAEMORRHAGIC FEVER
AND PRECIPITATION
IN FOUR PROVINCES OF THAILAND
1970–1979

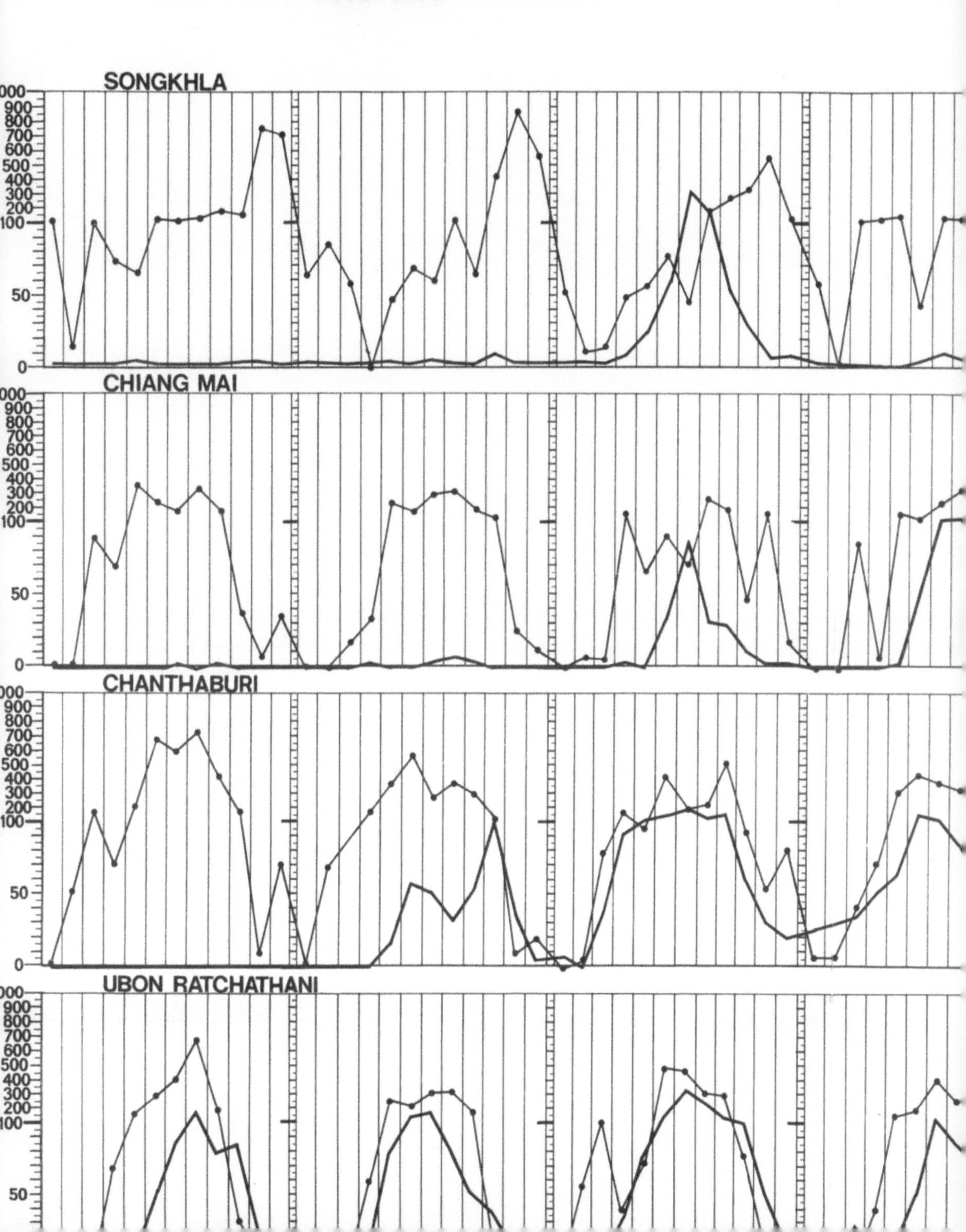

If you have any concerns about our products,
you can contact us on
ProductSafety@springernature.com

In case Publisher is established outside the EU,
the EU authorized representative is:
Springer Nature Customer Service Center GmbH
Europaplatz 3, 69115 Heidelberg, Germany

Printed by Libri Plureos GmbH
in Hamburg, Germany